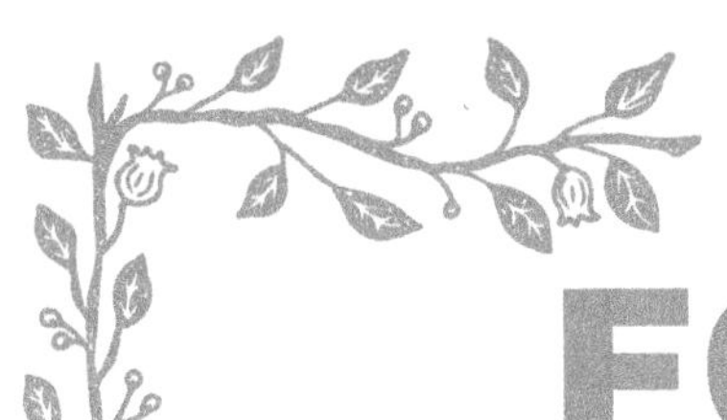

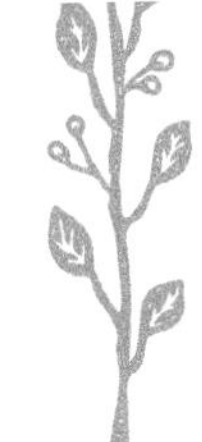

FOOD MENU

plant-based menopause

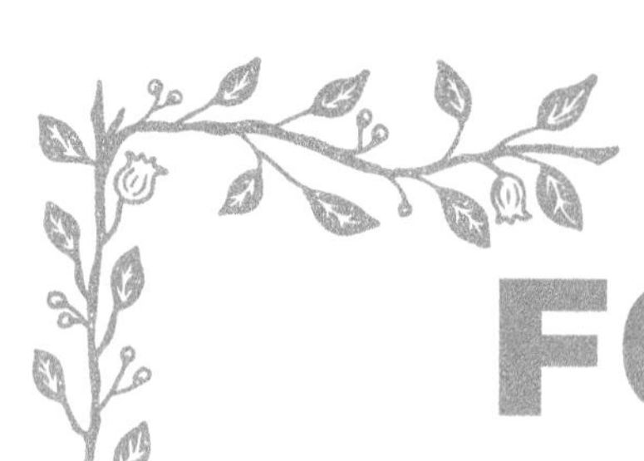

FOOD MENU
plant-based menopause

LUNCH

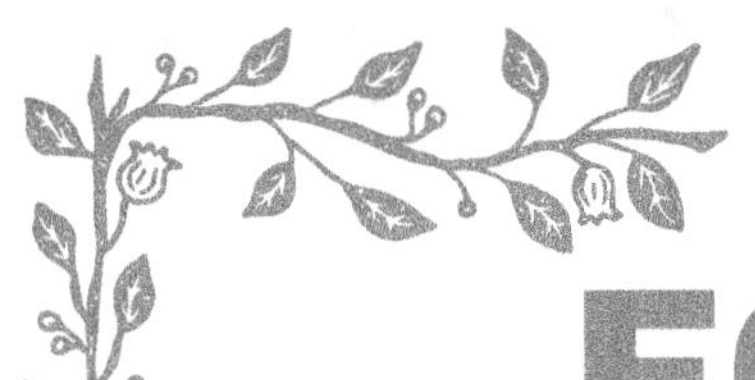

FOOD MENU

plant-based menopause

FOOD MENU

plant-based menopause

FOOD MENU

plant-based menopause

DESSERTS

1. Vegan Chocolate Avocado Mousse	84
2. Chia Seed Pudding with Mango	85
3. Baked Apples with Cinnamon	86
4. Vegan Banana Bread	87
5. Coconut Yogurt with Fresh Berries	88
6. Dark Chocolate and Nut Bark	89
7. Vegan Lemon Bars	90
8. Apple Crisp with Oat Topping	91
9. Vegan Chocolate Chip Cookies	92
10. Raspberry Chia Jam Bars	93

VEGETARIAN/VEGAN

2. Vegan Lentil Soup	94
3. Roasted Vegetable Medley	95
4. Vegan Tacos with Black Beans	96
5. Stuffed Eggplant with Quinoa	97
6. Vegan Mushroom Risotto	98
7. Chickpea and Spinach Stew	99
8. Vegan Vegetable Stir-Fry	100
9. Roasted Sweet Potato and Black Bean Burritos	101
10. Grilled Vegetable Kabobs	102

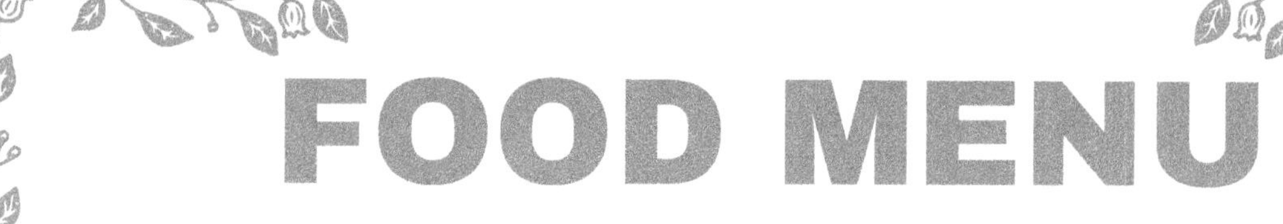

FOOD MENU

plant-based menopause

BEVERAGES

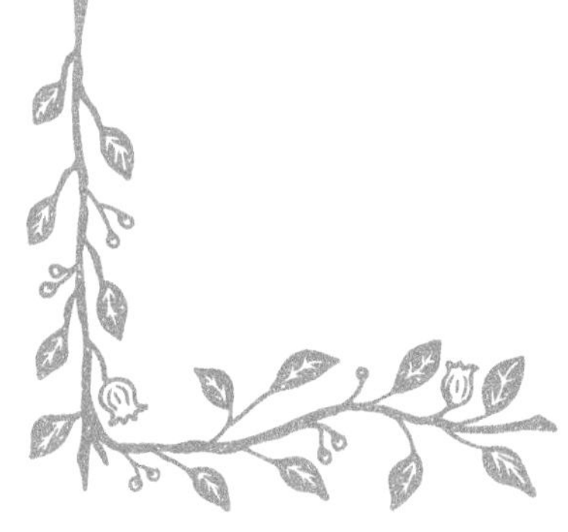

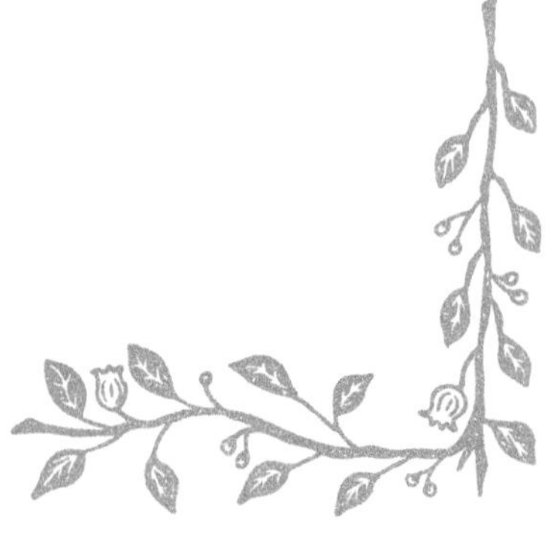

Welcome to the ***Plant-Based Menopause Cookbook: 110 Nutritious and Balanced Recipes for Managing Menopause.*** This cookbook is designed to provide you with delicious, nutrient-rich recipes to help manage the symptoms of menopause and promote overall well-being. By focusing on plant-based ingredients, you can enjoy meals that are both satisfying and beneficial for your health during this transitional phase of life.

Welcome to Plant-Based Eating

Eating a plant-based diet offers numerous benefits, especially during menopause. This approach emphasizes whole foods like fruits, vegetables, grains, nuts, seeds, and legumes, which are rich in essential nutrients and antioxidants. These foods can help manage menopause symptoms, support heart health, maintain a healthy weight, and improve overall energy levels.

Understanding Menopause

Menopause is a natural biological process that marks the end of a woman's menstrual cycles. It is diagnosed after 12 months without a menstrual period and usually occurs in the late 40s or early 50s. Menopause can bring about various symptoms, including hot flashes, night sweats, mood changes, and sleep disturbances. These symptoms are caused by changes in hormone levels, particularly estrogen and progesterone.

While menopause is a natural phase of life, managing its symptoms can be challenging. A balanced, plant-based diet can play a significant role in alleviating some of these symptoms and promoting a healthier lifestyle.

Nutritional Needs

During menopause, your body undergoes significant changes that can affect your nutritional needs. Incorporating the right nutrients into your diet is essential for managing symptoms and maintaining overall health:

- Phytoestrogens: These plant compounds mimic estrogen in the body and can help balance hormone levels. Foods rich in phytoestrogens include soy products, flaxseeds, and whole grains.

- Calcium and Vitamin D: These nutrients are crucial for bone health, which can be affected during menopause. Include sources like fortified plant milks, leafy greens, and almonds in your diet.

- Omega-3 Fatty Acids: Found in flaxseeds, chia seeds, walnuts, and algae-based supplements, omega-3s can help reduce inflammation and support heart health.

- Fiber: A high-fiber diet can help manage weight, improve digestion, and regulate blood sugar levels. Whole grains, fruits, vegetables, and legumes are excellent sources of fiber.

- Antioxidants: These compounds protect your cells from damage and support overall health. Berries, nuts, seeds, and colorful vegetables are rich in antioxidants.

Transitioning to Plant-Based

Switching to a plant-based diet may seem daunting at first, but with a few simple steps, you can make the transition smoothly and enjoy the benefits:

1. Start Gradually: Begin by incorporating more plant-based meals into your diet gradually. Replace one meal a day with a plant-based option and increase from there.

2. Plan Your Meals: Meal planning can help you stay on track and ensure you have all the ingredients you need for nutritious meals.

3. Experiment with New Recipes: Try out different recipes and ingredients to discover what you enjoy. This cookbook offers a wide variety of options to keep your meals exciting.

4. Focus on Whole Foods: Choose whole, minimally processed foods to maximize nutrient intake and health benefits.

5. Stay Hydrated: Drinking plenty of water is essential for overall health and can help manage menopause symptoms.

By embracing a plant-based diet, you are taking a significant step towards managing menopause symptoms and enhancing your overall health. This cookbook provides a diverse range of recipes to support you on this journey, from breakfast to dinner, snacks, and even desserts. Enjoy exploring these delicious, nutritious dishes and discover how plant-based eating can make a positive difference in your life during menopause.

1. Almond Butter and Banana Smoothie

PreparationTime: 5 minutes

Serves: 1

- 1 ripe banana, frozen
- 2 tbsp almond butter
- 1 cup unsweetened almond milk
- 1 tbsp honey (optional)
- 1/2 tsp vanilla extract
- Pinch of cinnamon (optional)

1. Add the frozen banana, almond butter, almond milk, honey (if using), vanilla extract, and cinnamon (if using) to a blender.

2. Blend on high speed until the mixture is smooth and creamy, about 1 minute.

3. Pour the almond butter and banana smoothie into a glass.

4. Serve immediately.

Tips:
- Use a ripe, frozen banana for a thick, creamy texture.
- Adjust the amount of almond milk to reach your desired consistency.
- Add a handful of spinach or kale for extra nutrients.
- Top with chopped almonds, shredded coconut, or a drizzle of extra almond butter.
- For a protein boost, add a scoop of vanilla protein powder.
- Substitute peanut butter or cashew butter for the almond butter.

This smoothie is a delicious and nutritious way to start your day. The combination of creamy almond butter, sweet banana, and nutty almond milk creates a rich, satisfying beverage. It's packed with healthy fats, fiber, and natural sweetness.

Enjoy this almond butter and banana smoothie as a quick breakfast or snack. It's sure to keep you feeling full and energized!

Breakfast

2. Chia Seed Pudding with Berries

PreparationTime: 10 minutes

Chilling Time: 2-4 hours

Serves: 2-3

- 1/4 cup chia seeds
- 1 cup unsweetened almond milk
- 2 tbsp maple syrup (or honey)
- 1 tsp vanilla extract
- 1 cup mixed berries (such as raspberries, blueberries, and strawberries)

Breakfast

1. In a medium bowl, whisk together the chia seeds, almond milk, maple syrup, and vanilla extract until well combined.

2. Cover the bowl and refrigerate for 2-4 hours, stirring occasionally, until the chia seeds have thickened the mixture into a pudding-like consistency.

3. Divide the chia seed pudding between serving bowls or jars.

4. Top each portion with the mixed berries.

5. Serve chilled.

Tips:
- For a thicker pudding, use 1/3 cup chia seeds.
- Substitute the almond milk with any milk of your choice.
- Try using different types of berries or fruit, such as mango, kiwi, or pineapple.
- Add a sprinkle of cinnamon, shredded coconut, or chopped nuts on top.
- Make the pudding in advance and store it in the refrigerator for up to 5 days.

Chia seed pudding is a delicious, nutrient-dense breakfast or snack. The chia seeds provide fiber, protein, and omega-3 fatty acids, while the berries add natural sweetness and antioxidants. This easy recipe makes a satisfying and healthy treat.

Enjoy this chia seed pudding with berries as a wholesome start to your day or as a refreshing dessert.

!

3. Quinoa Breakfast Bowl with Fruit

PreparationTime: 15 minutes

Cook Time: 15 minutes

Total Time: 30 minutes

Serves: 2

- 1/2 cup uncooked quinoa, rinsed
- 1 cup unsweetened almond milk
- 1 tsp vanilla extract
- 1/4 tsp ground cinnamon
- 1 tbsp maple syrup (optional)
- 1 cup mixed fresh fruit (such as berries, sliced banana, diced apple)
- 2 tbsp chopped nuts or seeds (such as almonds, walnuts, or chia seeds)

1. In a small saucepan, combine the rinsed quinoa and almond milk. Bring to a boil over medium-high heat.

2. Once boiling, reduce heat to low, cover and simmer for 12-15 minutes, until the quinoa is tender and the liquid is absorbed.

3. Remove from heat and stir in the vanilla extract, cinnamon, and maple syrup (if using).

4. Divide the cooked quinoa between two bowls.

5. Top each bowl with 1/2 cup of the mixed fresh fruit.

6. Sprinkle the chopped nuts or seeds over the top.

7. Serve the quinoa breakfast bowl warm or chilled.

Tips:
- Use any combination of your favorite fresh fruits.
- Substitute the almond milk with dairy milk, oat milk, or coconut milk.
- Add a spoonful of nut butter or a drizzle of honey for extra flavor.
- For a creamier texture, stir in a tablespoon of plain Greek yogurt.
- Make a larger batch of quinoa and store it in the fridge to use throughout the week.

This quinoa breakfast bowl is a nutritious and satisfying way to start your day. The protein-rich quinoa, fresh fruit, and crunchy nuts or seeds provide a balanced meal that will keep you feeling full and energized. Enjoy!

Breakfast

4. Spinach and Mushroom Tofu Scramble

PreparationTime: 10 minutes

Cook Time: 15 minutes

Total Time: 25 minutes

Serves: 2–3

- 1 block (14oz) extra-firm tofu, drained and crumbled
- 1 tbsp olive oil
- 8 oz cremini mushrooms, sliced
- 1 cup fresh spinach, chopped
- 2 cloves garlic, minced
- 1 tsp ground cumin
- 1 tsp turmeric
- 1/4 tsp cayenne pepper (optional)
- Salt and pepper to taste
- 2 tbsp nutritional yeast (optional)

1. In a large skillet, heat the olive oil over medium heat.

2. Add the sliced mushrooms and sauté for 5-7 minutes, until they start to brown.

3. Stir in the minced garlic and cook for 1 minute until fragrant.

4. Add the crumbled tofu, cumin, turmeric, cayenne (if using), salt, and pepper. Stir to combine.

5. Cook the tofu scramble for 5-7 minutes, stirring occasionally, until the tofu is heated through.

6. Stir in the chopped spinach and cook for 2-3 minutes until the spinach is wilted.

7. Remove from heat and stir in the nutritional yeast, if using.

8. Serve the spinach and mushroom tofu scramble warm, on its own or with toast, potatoes, or avocado.

Tips:
- Press the tofu for 30 minutes before crumbling to remove excess moisture.
- Use firm or extra-firm tofu for the best texture.
- Customize the spices to your taste - try adding paprika, oregano, or chili powder.
- For extra protein, stir in a tablespoon of peanut or almond butter.
- Garnish with chopped fresh herbs, diced tomatoes, or sliced avocado.

This savory tofu scramble is a delicious and nutritious plant-based breakfast or brunch option. The combination of protein-rich tofu, earthy mushrooms, and nutrient-dense spinach makes it a satisfying and flavorful meal.

Breakfast

5. Overnight Oats with Almond Milk and Apples

PreparationTime: 10 minutes
Chilling Time: 8 hours or overnight
Serves: 2

- 1 cup rolled oats
- 1 cup unsweetened almond milk
- 2 tbsp chia seeds
- 1 tbsp maple syrup (or honey)
- 1/2 tsp ground cinnamon
- 1 medium apple, diced
- 2 tbsp chopped walnuts (optional)

1. In a medium bowl or mason jar, combine the rolled oats, almond milk, chia seeds, maple syrup, and cinnamon. Stir well to mix.

2. Cover the bowl or seal the mason jar and refrigerate for at least 8 hours, or overnight.

3. In the morning, remove the overnight oats from the fridge. Stir in the diced apple.

4. Top the oats with the chopped walnuts, if using.

5. Serve the overnight oats chilled.

Tips:
- Use any type of milk you prefer - dairy, oat, or coconut milk all work well.
- Substitute the maple syrup with honey, agave, or your favorite sweetener.
- Try different fruit combinations like berries, bananas, or pears.
- Add a spoonful of nut butter or a sprinkle of cinnamon or nutmeg for extra flavor.
- Make a larger batch and store individual servings in the fridge for easy grab-and-go breakfasts.

Overnight oats are a simple, make-ahead breakfast that's packed with fiber, protein, and nutrients. The combination of creamy almond milk, crunchy apples, and nutty walnuts makes this a delicious and satisfying morning meal.

Enjoy this easy overnight oats recipe as a healthy start to your day!

Breakfast

6. Sweet Potato and Black Bean Breakfast Burrito

PreparationTime: 15 minutes

Cook Time: 20 minutes

Total Time: 35 minutes

Serves: 4 burritos

- 1 medium sweet potato, peeled and diced
- 1 tbsp olive oil
- 1 (15oz) can black beans, drained and rinsed
- 4 large eggs, scrambled
- 1/2 cup shredded cheddar cheese
- 4 whole wheat tortillas
- Salt and pepper to taste
- Optional toppings: salsa, avocado, hot sauce

Breakfast

1. In a skillet, heat the olive oil over medium heat. Add the diced sweet potato and sauté for 12-15 minutes, until tender.

2. Stir the black beans into the cooked sweet potatoes and heat through, about 2-3 minutes.

3. In a separate skillet, scramble the eggs until cooked through.

4. To assemble the burritos, lay out the tortillas and divide the sweet potato-black bean mixture evenly among them. Top each with the scrambled eggs and shredded cheese.

5. Fold the bottom of the tortilla up, then fold in the sides and roll up tightly to create a burrito.

6. Serve the breakfast burritos warm, with desired toppings like salsa, avocado, or hot sauce.

Tips:
- Roast the sweet potato cubes in the oven at 400°F for 15-20 minutes if you prefer.
- Add diced bell peppers, onions, or spinach to the sweet potato mixture.
- Use a different type of cheese, such as pepper jack or feta.
- Wrap the burritos individually in foil or parchment paper for easy grab-and-go meals.
- Freeze the assembled burritos for up to 3 months. Reheat in the microwave or oven when ready to eat.

These sweet potato and black bean breakfast burritos are a nutritious and satisfying way to start your day. The combination of roasted sweet potatoes, protein-packed black beans, and fluffy scrambled eggs makes for a delicious and filling breakfast.

Enjoy these burritos as a wholesome on-the-go breakfast option!

7. Blueberry and Flaxseed Pancakes

PreparationTime: 10 minutes

Cook Time: 15 minutes

Total Time: 25 minutes

Serves: 4 (makes 8 pancakes)

- 1 cup whole wheat flour
- 2 tbsp ground flaxseed
- 1 tsp baking powder
- 1/4 tsp baking soda
- 1/4 tsp salt
- 1 cup unsweetened almond milk
- 1 egg
- 1 tbsp maple syrup
- 1 tsp vanilla extract
- 1 cup fresh or frozen blueberries

Breakfast

1. In a medium bowl, whisk together the whole wheat flour, ground flaxseed, baking powder, baking soda, and salt.

2. In a separate bowl, whisk the almond milk, egg, maple syrup, and vanilla extract until well combined.

3. Pour the wet ingredients into the dry ingredients and stir just until combined (do not overmix).

4. Gently fold in the blueberries.

5. Heat a lightly oiled skillet or griddle over medium heat.

6. Scoop 1/4 cup portions of the batter onto the hot surface, cooking for 2-3 minutes per side until golden brown.

7. Serve the blueberry flaxseed pancakes warm, with additional maple syrup, fresh blueberries, or your favorite toppings.

Tips:
- Use fresh or frozen blueberries. If using frozen, do not thaw them first.
- Substitute the whole wheat flour with all-purpose or gluten-free flour.
- Add a tablespoon of chia seeds or chopped walnuts for extra nutrition.
- Top the pancakes with sliced bananas, a dollop of Greek yogurt, or a sprinkle of cinnamon.
- Make a larger batch and reheat leftovers in the toaster or microwave for quick breakfasts.

These blueberry and flaxseed pancakes are a delicious and nutritious way to start your day. The whole wheat flour, flaxseed, and fresh blueberries provide fiber, protein, and antioxidants to keep you feeling full and energized.

Enjoy these healthy pancakes for a satisfying breakfast!

8. Avocado Toast with Tomato and Basil

PreparationTime: 10 minutes
Cook Time: 0 minutes
Total Time: 10 minutes
Serves: 2

- 2 slices whole grain bread, toasted
- 1 ripe avocado, mashed
- 1 tomato, diced
- 2 tbsp fresh basil leaves, chopped
- 1 tbsp olive oil
- 1 tsp balsamic glaze (optional)
- Salt and pepper to taste

Breakfast

1. Toast the bread slices until golden brown.

2. In a small bowl, mash the avocado with a fork until smooth.

3. Spread the mashed avocado evenly over the toasted bread slices.

4. Top the avocado toast with the diced tomatoes and chopped basil leaves.

5. Drizzle the olive oil over the top.

6. If desired, drizzle a small amount of balsamic glaze over the toast.

7. Season with salt and pepper to taste.

8. Serve immediately.

Nutrition Information (per serving):
Calories: 250
Fat: 16g
Carbohydrates: 22g
Fiber: 8g
Protein: 5g
Vitamin C: 20% DV
Potassium: 15% DV

This avocado toast makes for a delicious and nutritious breakfast or snack. The creamy avocado, juicy tomatoes, and fragrant basil create a flavorful and satisfying combination.

9. Vegan Protein Pancakes

PreparationTime: 10 minutes

Cook Time: 10 minutes

Total Time: 20 minutes

Serves: 4 (makes 8 pancakes)

- 1 cup all-purpose flour
- 1/2 cup rolled oats
- 2 scoops (about 1/2 cup) vanilla protein powder
- 2 tsp baking powder
- 1/4 tsp salt
- 1 cup unsweetened almond milk
- 2 tbsp maple syrup
- 1 tsp vanilla extract

Toppings (optional):
- Fresh berries
- Sliced bananas
- Chopped nuts
- Maple syrup

Breakfast

1. In a large bowl, whisk together the flour, rolled oats, protein powder, baking powder, and salt.

2. In a separate bowl, combine the almond milk, maple syrup, and vanilla extract.

3. Pour the wet ingredients into the dry ingredients and stir just until combined (do not overmix).

4. Heat a lightly oiled non-stick skillet or griddle over medium heat.

5. Scoop about 1/4 cup of the batter onto the hot surface and cook for 2-3 minutes per side, or until golden brown.

6. Repeat with the remaining batter, keeping the cooked pancakes warm in a 200°F oven.

7. Serve the vegan protein pancakes warm, topped with your desired toppings.

Nutrition Information (per serving, 2 pancakes):
Calories: 260
Protein: 18g
Fat: 5g
Carbohydrates: 40g
Fiber: 4g

These vegan protein pancakes are a great way to start your day with a nutritious and filling breakfast. The combination of protein powder, oats, and almond milk provides a boost of protein and fiber to keep you satisfied.

10. Green Smoothie Bowl with Kiwi and Hemp Seeds

PreparationTime: 5 minutes

Cook Time: 0 minutes

Total Time: 5 minutes

Serves: 1

- 1 cup spinach or kale, packed
- 1 cup unsweetened almond milk
- 1 banana, frozen
- 1 kiwi, peeled and chopped
- 2 tbsp hemp seeds
- 1 tbsp honey or maple syrup (optional)

Breakfast

1. In a high-speed blender, combine the spinach/kale, almond milk, and frozen banana. Blend until smooth and creamy.

2. Pour the smoothie into a bowl.

3. Top with the chopped kiwi and hemp seeds.

4. Drizzle with honey or maple syrup if desired.

5. Enjoy immediately with a spoon.

Nutrition Information (per serving):
Calories: 300
Protein: 10g
Fat: 12g
Carbohydrates: 44g
Fiber: 8g
Vitamin C: 70% DV
Vitamin K: 200% DV

This green smoothie bowl is a nutritious and delicious way to start your day. The combination of leafy greens, fruit, and healthy fats from the hemp seeds provides a balanced and satisfying meal.

11. Vegan French Toast with Berries

PreparationTime: 15 minutes

Cook Time: 10 minutes

Total Time: 25 minutes

Serves: 4 (makes 8 slices of french toast)

- 8 slices of thick-cut bread (use a sturdy, crusty bread)
- 1 cup unsweetened almond milk
- 1/4 cup chickpea flour (or all-purpose flour)
- 2 tbsp maple syrup
- 1 tsp vanilla extract
- 1/2 tsp ground cinnamon
- 1/4 tsp ground nutmeg
- 1 cup mixed berries (such as strawberries, blueberries, raspberries)
- Coconut oil or vegan butter for cooking

Toppings (optional):
- Powdered sugar
- Additional maple syrup
- Chopped nuts

Breakfast

1. In a shallow bowl, whisk together the almond milk, chickpea flour, maple syrup, vanilla, cinnamon, and nutmeg until well combined.

2. Dip the bread slices into the batter, coating both sides evenly.

3. Heat a large non-stick skillet or griddle over medium heat and grease with a small amount of coconut oil or vegan butter.

4. Cook the battered bread slices for 2-3 minutes per side, or until golden brown.

5. Transfer the cooked french toast slices to a plate and keep warm in a 200°F oven while you cook the remaining slices.

6. Serve the vegan french toast warm, topped with the mixed berries and any desired toppings.

Nutrition Information (per serving, 2 slices):
Calories: 280
Protein: 8g
Fat: 8g
Carbohydrates: 44g
Fiber: 5g
Vitamin C: 25% DV

This vegan french toast is a delicious and nutritious breakfast option. The chickpea flour and almond milk create a custard-like batter, while the berries add a fresh and fruity element.

12. Oatmeal with Pumpkin Seeds and Maple Syrup

PreparationTime: 5 minutes

Cook Time: 10 minutes

Total Time: 15 minutes

Serves: 2

- 1 cup old-fashioned rolled oats
- 2 cups unsweetened almond milk (or milk of your choice)
- 1/4 tsp ground cinnamon
- 1/8 tsp ground nutmeg
- 2 tbsp pumpkin seeds
- 2 tbsp pure maple syrup
- 1 tbsp chopped walnuts (optional)

Breakfast

1. In a medium saucepan, combine the rolled oats and almond milk. Bring to a simmer over medium heat, stirring occasionally.

2. Once the oats have thickened to your desired consistency, about 5-7 minutes, remove from heat.

3. Stir in the ground cinnamon and nutmeg.

4. Transfer the oatmeal to two serving bowls.

5. Top each bowl with 1 tbsp of pumpkin seeds and 1 tbsp of maple syrup.

6. If desired, sprinkle 1/2 tbsp of chopped walnuts over each bowl.

7. Serve warm.

Nutrition Information (per serving):
Calories: 280
Protein: 8g
Fat: 10g
Carbohydrates: 41g
Fiber: 6g
Vitamin A: 2% DV
Vitamin C: 2% DV

This oatmeal dish is a nutritious and satisfying breakfast. The pumpkin seeds provide a boost of protein, healthy fats, and minerals, while the maple syrup adds a touch of natural sweetness. The cinnamon and nutmeg provide a cozy, autumnal flavor.

13. Tropical Fruit Parfait with Coconut Yogurt

PreparationTime: 15 minutes

Cook Time: 0 minutes

Total Time: 15 minutes

Serves: 2

- 1 cup plain coconut yogurt
- 1 cup diced pineapple
- 1 cup diced mango
- 1/2 cup diced kiwi
- 2 tbsp toasted coconut flakes
- 1 tbsp honey (optional)

Breakfast

1. In two parfait glasses or small bowls, layer the ingredients in the following order:
   - 1/4 cup coconut yogurt
   - 1/4 cup diced pineapple
   - 1/4 cup diced mango
   - 1/4 cup diced kiwi
   - Repeat the layers

2. Top each parfait with 1 tbsp of toasted coconut flakes.

3. If desired, drizzle 1/2 tbsp of honey over each parfait.

4. Serve chilled.

Nutrition Information (per serving):
Calories: 200
Protein: 5g
Fat: 6g
Carbohydrates: 34g
Fiber: 4g
Vitamin C: 100% DV
Potassium: 15% DV

This tropical fruit parfait is a refreshing and healthy dessert or snack. The creamy coconut yogurt pairs perfectly with the sweet and juicy pineapple, mango, and kiwi. The toasted coconut flakes add a nice crunch and texture.

14. Vegan Breakfast Tacos

PreparationTime: 15 minutes

Cook Time: 15 minutes

Total Time: 30 minutes

Serves: 4 (makes 8 tacos)

- 8 small corn or flour tortillas
- 1 block (14 oz) extra-firm tofu, crumbled
- 1 tbsp olive oil
- 1 tsp ground cumin
- 1 tsp chili powder
- 1/2 tsp garlic powder
- Salt and pepper to taste
- 1 cup diced bell peppers (any color)
- 1/2 cup diced onion
- 1 avocado, sliced
- 2 tbsp chopped fresh cilantro
- 1 lime, cut into wedges

Breakfast

1. Heat the olive oil in a large skillet over medium heat. Add the crumbled tofu, cumin, chili powder, garlic powder, salt, and pepper. Cook for 5-7 minutes, stirring occasionally, until the tofu is lightly browned.

2. Add the diced bell peppers and onion to the skillet. Cook for an additional 5-7 minutes, or until the vegetables are tender.

3. Warm the tortillas according to package Directions.

4. To assemble the tacos, place a spoonful of the tofu and vegetable mixture into each tortilla. Top with sliced avocado and chopped cilantro.

5. Serve the vegan breakfast tacos immediately, with lime wedges on the side for squeezing over the top.

Nutrition Information (per serving, 2 tacos):
Calories: 320
Protein: 12g
Fat: 16g
Carbohydrates: 36g
Fiber: 8g
Vitamin C: 60% DV
Potassium: 15% DV

These vegan breakfast tacos are a delicious and satisfying way to start your day. The crumbled tofu provides a protein-rich filling, while the fresh vegetables and avocado add flavor and nutrition.

15. Apple Cinnamon Breakfast Quinoa

PreparationTime: 10 minutes
Cook Time: 20 minutes
Total Time: 30 minutes
Serves: 4

- 1 cup uncooked quinoa, rinsed
- 2 cups unsweetened almond milk
- 1 apple, peeled, cored, and diced
- 2 tbsp maple syrup
- 1 tsp ground cinnamon
- 1/4 tsp ground nutmeg
- 1/4 tsp salt
- 2 tbsp chopped walnuts (optional)

Breakfast

1. In a medium saucepan, combine the rinsed quinoa and almond milk. Bring to a boil over medium-high heat.

2. Once boiling, reduce the heat to low, cover, and simmer for 15-20 minutes, or until the quinoa is cooked and the liquid is absorbed.

3. Remove the saucepan from the heat and stir in the diced apple, maple syrup, cinnamon, nutmeg, and salt.

4. Serve the apple cinnamon breakfast quinoa warm, topped with the chopped walnuts (if using).

Nutrition Information (per serving):
Calories: 220
Protein: 6g
Fat: 5g
Carbohydrates: 38g
Fiber: 4g
Vitamin A: 2% DV
Vitamin C: 4% DV

This Apple Cinnamon Breakfast Quinoa is a delicious and nutritious way to start your day. The quinoa provides a good source of protein and fiber, while the apples, cinnamon, and maple syrup create a comforting and flavorful dish. It's a great alternative to traditional oatmeal or porridge.

1. Chickpea and Avocado Salad

PreparationTime: 15 minutes

Cook Time: 0 minutes

Total Time: 15 minutes

Serves: 4

- 1 (15 oz) can chickpeas, drained and rinsed
- 1 ripe avocado, diced
- 1/2 cup diced cucumber
- 1/4 cup diced red onion
- 2 tbsp chopped fresh cilantro
- 2 tbsp fresh lemon juice
- 1 tbsp olive oil
- 1/2 tsp ground cumin
- Salt and pepper to taste

1. In a large bowl, combine the drained and rinsed chickpeas, diced avocado, cucumber, red onion, and chopped cilantro.

2. In a small bowl, whisk together the lemon juice, olive oil, and ground cumin.

3. Pour the dressing over the chickpea and avocado mixture and gently toss to coat.

4. Season with salt and pepper to taste.

5. Serve immediately or refrigerate until ready to serve.

Nutrition Information (per serving):
Calories: 180
Protein: 6g
Fat: 10g
Carbohydrates: 18g
Fiber: 7g
Vitamin C: 15% DV
Potassium: 20% DV

This Chickpea and Avocado Salad is a nutritious and flavorful dish that can be enjoyed as a main course, side salad, or even as a dip with crackers or pita bread. The combination of protein-rich chickpeas, creamy avocado, and fresh vegetables makes it a satisfying and versatile option.

Lunch

2. Quinoa and Roasted Vegetable Salad

PreparationTime: 20 minutes
Cook Time: 30 minutes
Total Time: 50 minutes
Serves: 4

- 1 cup uncooked quinoa, rinsed
- 2 cups vegetable broth
- 1 medium zucchini, diced
- 1 red bell pepper, diced
- 1 cup diced butternut squash
- 1 red onion, diced
- 2 tbsp olive oil
- 1 tsp dried thyme
- Salt and pepper to taste
- 2 tbsp balsamic vinegar
- 2 tbsp chopped fresh parsley

Lunch

1. Preheat the oven to 400°F (200°C).

2. In a medium saucepan, combine the quinoa and vegetable broth. Bring to a boil, then reduce heat to low, cover, and simmer for 15-20 minutes, or until the quinoa is cooked and the liquid is absorbed. Fluff with a fork and set aside.

3. On a large baking sheet, toss the diced zucchini, bell pepper, butternut squash, and red onion with the olive oil, dried thyme, salt, and pepper.

4. Roast the vegetables in the preheated oven for 25-30 minutes, or until they are tender and lightly browned, stirring halfway through.

5. In a large bowl, combine the cooked quinoa and roasted vegetables.

6. Drizzle the balsamic vinegar over the salad and gently toss to coat.

7. Garnish with the chopped fresh parsley.

8. Serve warm or at room temperature.

Nutrition Information (per serving):
Calories: 280
Protein: 8g
Fat: 9g
Carbohydrates: 42g
Fiber: 6g
Vitamin A: 25% DV
Vitamin C: 80% DV

This Quinoa and Roasted Vegetable Salad is a nutritious and flavorful dish that can be enjoyed as a main course or a side. The combination of fluffy quinoa and roasted vegetables, dressed with a balsamic vinaigrette, makes for a satisfying and versatile meal.

3. Vegan Caesar Salad with Crispy Chickpeas

PreparationTime: 20 minutes

Cook Time: 20 minutes

Total Time: 40 minutes

Serves: 4

For the Crispy Chickpeas:
- 1 (15 oz) can chickpeas, drained and rinsed
- 1 tbsp olive oil
- 1 tsp garlic powder
- 1/2 tsp onion powder
- 1/4 tsp salt

For the Vegan Caesar Dressing:
- 1/2 cup raw cashews, soaked in water for at least 4 hours or overnight
- 1/4 cup water
- 2 tbsp lemon juice
- 2 tbsp Dijon mustard
- 1 garlic clove, minced
- 1 tsp Worcestershire sauce (use vegan Worcestershire)
- 1/4 tsp salt

For the Salad:
- 1 head romaine lettuce, chopped
- 1/2 cup cherry tomatoes, halved
- 2 tbsp chopped fresh parsley

Lunch

1. Preheat the oven to 400°F (200°C). Drain and rinse the chickpeas, then pat them dry with a paper towel. Toss the chickpeas with the olive oil, garlic powder, onion powder, and salt. Spread them on a baking sheet and roast for 15-20 minutes, shaking the pan halfway, until crispy.

2. In a high-speed blender, combine the soaked and drained cashews, water, lemon juice, Dijon mustard, garlic, Worcestershire sauce, and salt. Blend until smooth and creamy. Taste and adjust seasoning as needed.

3. In a large salad bowl, combine the chopped romaine lettuce, cherry tomatoes, and parsley.

4. Drizzle the vegan Caesar dressing over the salad and toss to coat.

5. Top the salad with the crispy chickpeas.

6. Serve immediately.

Nutrition Information (per serving):
Calories: 280
Protein: 10g
Fat: 16g
Carbohydrates: 24g
Fiber: 7g
Vitamin A: 120% DV
Vitamin C: 25% DV

This Vegan Caesar Salad with Crispy Chickpeas is a delicious and nutritious twist on the classic Caesar salad. The creamy cashew-based dressing and the crunchy roasted chickpeas make this a satisfying and flavorful plant-based meal.

4. Lentil and Spinach Soup

PreparationTime: 15 minutes

Cook Time: 30 minutes

Total Time: 45 minutes

Serves: 4

- 1 tbsp olive oil
- 1 onion, diced
- 3 garlic cloves, minced
- 1 cup dried brown or green lentils, rinsed
- 4 cups vegetable broth
- 1 (14 oz) can diced tomatoes
- 1 tsp ground cumin
- 1 tsp dried oregano
- 1/4 tsp red pepper flakes (optional)
- Salt and pepper to taste
- 4 cups fresh spinach, chopped
- 2 tbsp chopped fresh parsley

Lunch

1. In a large pot or Dutch oven, heat the olive oil over medium heat. Add the diced onion and sauté for 5 minutes, until translucent.

2. Add the minced garlic and sauté for an additional minute, until fragrant.

3. Stir in the rinsed lentils, vegetable broth, diced tomatoes, cumin, oregano, and red pepper flakes (if using). Season with salt and pepper.

4. Bring the soup to a boil, then reduce the heat to low, cover, and simmer for 20-25 minutes, or until the lentils are tender.

5. Stir in the chopped spinach and continue to cook for 2-3 minutes, until the spinach is wilted.

6. Remove the soup from heat and stir in the chopped fresh parsley.

7. Serve the lentil and spinach soup hot, with crusty bread or crackers on the side.

Nutrition Information (per serving):
Calories: 250
Protein: 15g
Fat: 5g
Carbohydrates: 35g
Fiber: 12g
Vitamin A: 50% DV
Vitamin C: 20% DV

This Lentil and Spinach Soup is a hearty, nutritious, and flavorful dish. The combination of protein-rich lentils, nutrient-dense spinach, and aromatic spices makes it a satisfying and comforting meal.

5. Mediterranean Buddha Bowl

PreparationTime: 20 minutes
Cook Time: 20 minutes
Total Time: 40 minutes
Serves: 4

- 1 cup uncooked quinoa, rinsed
- 2 cups vegetable broth
- 1 cup diced cucumber
- 1 cup cherry tomatoes, halved
- 1 cup cooked chickpeas
- 1/2 cup crumbled feta cheese
- 1/4 cup kalamata olives, sliced
- 2 tbsp chopped fresh parsley
- 2 tbsp olive oil
- 2 tbsp lemon juice
- 1 tsp dried oregano
- Salt and pepper to taste

1. In a medium saucepan, combine the quinoa and vegetable broth. Bring to a boil, then reduce heat to low, cover, and simmer for 15-20 minutes, or until the quinoa is cooked and the liquid is absorbed.

2. In a large bowl, combine the cooked quinoa, diced cucumber, cherry tomatoes, chickpeas, feta cheese, and sliced olives.

3. In a small bowl, whisk together the olive oil, lemon juice, dried oregano, salt, and pepper.

4. Drizzle the dressing over the quinoa and vegetable mixture and gently toss to coat.

5. Garnish with the chopped fresh parsley.

6. Serve immediately or refrigerate until ready to serve.

Nutrition Information (per serving):
Calories: 350
Protein: 12g
Fat: 16g
Carbohydrates: 40g
Fiber: 7g
Vitamin A: 15% DV
Vitamin C: 20% DV

This Mediterranean Buddha Bowl is a nutritious and flavorful meal that combines the nutty quinoa, fresh vegetables, protein-rich chickpeas, and tangy feta cheese. The lemon-oregano dressing ties all the flavors together for a delicious and satisfying dish.

Lunch

6. Grilled Vegetable and Hummus Wrap

PreparationTime: 20 minutes
Cook Time: 15 minutes
Total Time: 35 minutes
Serves: 4

- 1 zucchini, sliced lengthwise into 1/4-inch thick strips
- 1 red bell pepper, sliced into strips
- 1 yellow squash, sliced lengthwise into 1/4-inch thick strips
- 1 red onion, sliced into 1/2-inch thick rings
- 2 tbsp olive oil
- Salt and pepper to taste
- 4 whole wheat tortillas or wraps
- 1 cup hummus
- 1 cup baby spinach or arugula
- 1/4 cup crumbled feta cheese (optional)

Lunch

1. Preheat a grill or grill pan over medium-high heat.

2. In a large bowl, toss the zucchini, bell pepper, yellow squash, and red onion slices with the olive oil. Season with salt and pepper.

3. Grill the vegetables for 2-3 minutes per side, or until they are tender and have grill marks.

4. Remove the grilled vegetables from the heat and let them cool slightly.

5. Spread about 1/4 cup of hummus onto each tortilla or wrap, leaving a 1-inch border.

6. Arrange the grilled vegetables in a line down the center of the tortilla.

7. Top the vegetables with a handful of baby spinach or arugula.

8. If using, sprinkle the crumbled feta cheese over the top.

9. Fold the bottom of the tortilla up over the filling, then fold in the sides and continue rolling tightly to create a wrap.

10. Serve the grilled vegetable and hummus wraps immediately.

Nutrition Information (per serving):
Calories: 350
Protein: 10g
Fat: 16g
Carbohydrates: 43g
Fiber: 7g
Vitamin A: 50% DV
Vitamin C: 70% DV

7. Vegan Sushi Rolls with Tofu

PreparationTime: 30 minutes

Cook Time: 20 minutes

Total Time: 50 minutes

Serves: 4 (makes 8 rolls)

- 1 cup uncooked short-grain brown rice
- 2 cups water
- 1/4 cup rice vinegar
- 1 tbsp maple syrup
- 1/2 tsp salt
- 1 block (14 oz) extra-firm tofu, pressed and cut into thin strips
- 2 tbsp low-sodium soy sauce or tamari
- 1 tsp sesame oil
- 1 avocado, sliced
- 1 cucumber, peeled and cut into thin strips
- 1 carrot, peeled and cut into thin strips
- 8 sheets of nori (seaweed sheets)
- Wasabi and pickled ginger, for serving (optional)

1. Cook the brown rice: In a medium saucepan, combine the rice and water. Bring to a boil, then reduce heat to low, cover, and simmer for 20 minutes, or until the rice is tender and the water is absorbed. Fluff with a fork and set aside.

2. In a small bowl, whisk together the rice vinegar, maple syrup, and salt. Add the cooked rice and gently toss to coat. Set aside.

3. In a shallow dish, combine the tofu strips, soy sauce, and sesame oil. Marinate for 10-15 minutes.

4. Lay a nori sheet shiny-side down on a bamboo sushi mat or clean work surface. Spread about 1/2 cup of the seasoned rice evenly over the nori, leaving a 1-inch border at the top.

5. Arrange a few strips of tofu, avocado, cucumber, and carrot in a line across the center of the rice.

6. Carefully roll the nori around the fillings, using the bamboo mat to help you roll tightly. Moisten the top edge of the nori with water to seal the roll.

7. Repeat with the remaining nori sheets and fillings.

8. Slice each roll into 4-6 pieces using a sharp knife.

9. Serve the vegan sushi rolls with wasabi and pickled ginger, if desired.

Nutrition Information (per serving, 2 rolls):
Calories: 320
Protein: 12g
Fat: 12g
Carbohydrates: 44g
Fiber: 6g
Vitamin A: 60% DV
Vitamin C: 15% DV

8. Spicy Black Bean Soup

PreparationTime: 15 minutes

Cook Time: 30 minutes

Total Time: 45 minutes

Serves: 4

- 2 tbsp olive oil
- 1 onion, diced
- 3 garlic cloves, minced
- 2 tsp ground cumin
- 1 tsp chili powder
- 1/2 tsp smoked paprika
- 1/4 tsp cayenne pepper (or to taste)
- 2 (15 oz) cans black beans, drained and rinsed
- 4 cups vegetable broth
- 1 (14 oz) can diced tomatoes
- 1 tsp dried oregano
- Salt and pepper to taste
- Chopped fresh cilantro for garnish
- Lime wedges for serving

Lunch

1. In a large pot or Dutch oven, heat the olive oil over medium heat. Add the diced onion and sauté for 5-7 minutes, until translucent.

2. Add the minced garlic, cumin, chili powder, smoked paprika, and cayenne pepper. Cook for 1-2 minutes, stirring constantly, until fragrant.

3. Stir in the drained and rinsed black beans, vegetable broth, diced tomatoes, and dried oregano. Season with salt and pepper to taste.

4. Bring the soup to a boil, then reduce the heat to low and let it simmer for 20-25 minutes, stirring occasionally, until the flavors have melded and the soup has thickened slightly.

5. Taste and adjust seasoning as needed.

6. Ladle the spicy black bean soup into bowls and garnish with chopped fresh cilantro.

7. Serve with lime wedges on the side for squeezing over the top.

Nutrition Information (per serving):
Calories: 280
Protein: 12g
Fat: 7g
Carbohydrates: 42g
Fiber: 12g
Vitamin A: 10% DV
Vitamin C: 15% DV

This Spicy Black Bean Soup is a comforting and flavorful plant-based meal. The combination of black beans, diced tomatoes, and aromatic spices creates a satisfying and nutritious soup that's perfect for a cozy dinner.

9. Stuffed Bell Peppers with Quinoa and Black Beans

PreparationTime: 20 minutes

Cook Time: 40 minutes

Total Time: 1 hour

Serves: 4 (makes 8 stuffed pepper halves)

- 4 bell peppers, halved lengthwise and seeds removed
- 1 cup cooked quinoa
- 1 (15 oz) can black beans, drained and rinsed
- 1 cup diced tomatoes
- 1/2 cup diced onion
- 2 garlic cloves, minced
- 1 tsp ground cumin
- 1 tsp chili powder
- 1/4 tsp smoked paprika
- Salt and pepper to taste
- 1/2 cup shredded vegan cheddar cheese (optional)
- Chopped fresh cilantro for garnish

1. Preheat the oven to 375°F (190°C).

2. Arrange the bell pepper halves in a baking dish or on a rimmed baking sheet.

3. In a large bowl, combine the cooked quinoa, black beans, diced tomatoes, onion, garlic, cumin, chili powder, smoked paprika, salt, and pepper. Mix well.

4. Spoon the quinoa and black bean mixture evenly into the bell pepper halves.

5. If using, sprinkle the shredded vegan cheddar cheese over the top of the stuffed peppers.

6. Bake for 35-40 minutes, or until the peppers are tender and the filling is hot.

7. Remove the stuffed peppers from the oven and garnish with chopped fresh cilantro.

8. Serve warm.

Nutrition Information (per serving, 2 stuffed pepper halves):
Calories: 280
Protein: 12g
Fat: 4g
Carbohydrates: 48g
Fiber: 12g
Vitamin A: 60% DV
Vitamin C: 150% DV

These Stuffed Bell Peppers with Quinoa and Black Beans are a delicious and nutritious plant-based meal. The combination of protein-rich quinoa and black beans, along with the flavorful spices, makes for a satisfying and wholesome dish.

10. Thai Peanut Noodle Salad

PreparationTime: 20 minutes

Cook Time: 10 minutes

Total Time: 30 minutes

Serves: 4

- 8 oz whole wheat spaghetti or rice noodles
- 1/2 cup creamy peanut butter
- 3 tbsp low-sodium soy sauce
- 2 tbsp rice vinegar
- 1 tbsp honey or maple syrup
- 1 tsp sesame oil
- 1 tsp grated fresh ginger
- 1 garlic clove, minced
- 1/4 tsp red pepper flakes (optional)
- 1 cup shredded cabbage
- 1 cup shredded carrots
- 1/2 cup chopped fresh cilantro
- 2 tbsp chopped roasted peanuts
- 1 lime, cut into wedges

1. Cook the spaghetti or rice noodles according to package Directions. Drain and rinse under cold water to cool.

2. In a medium bowl, whisk together the peanut butter, soy sauce, rice vinegar, honey, sesame oil, grated ginger, garlic, and red pepper flakes (if using).

3. Add the cooked and cooled noodles, shredded cabbage, shredded carrots, and chopped cilantro to the peanut sauce. Toss to coat everything evenly.

4. Transfer the Thai peanut noodle salad to a serving bowl or plate.

5. Sprinkle the chopped roasted peanuts over the top.

6. Serve the salad immediately, with lime wedges on the side for squeezing over the top.

Nutrition Information (per serving):
Calories: 350
Protein: 12g
Fat: 15g
Carbohydrates: 44g
Fiber: 6g
Vitamin A: 100% DV
Vitamin C: 15% DV

This Thai Peanut Noodle Salad is a delicious and nutritious plant-based meal. The creamy peanut sauce, crunchy vegetables, and chewy noodles make for a satisfying and flavorful dish.

Lunch

11. Vegan BLT Sandwich

PreparationTime: 15 minutes

Cook Time: 15 minutes

Total Time: 30 minutes

Serves: 2

- 4 slices of toasted whole grain bread
- 4 slices of vegan bacon (such as tempeh or coconut bacon)
- 1 tomato, sliced
- 1 cup shredded lettuce
- 2 tbsp vegan mayonnaise
- Salt and pepper to taste

Lunch

1. Cook the vegan bacon according to package Directions, or make your own homemade coconut bacon. Set aside.

2. Toast the whole grain bread slices until golden brown.

3. Spread 1 tbsp of vegan mayonnaise on each of the 4 toast slices.

4. Layer the vegan bacon, tomato slices, and shredded lettuce on 2 of the toast slices.

5. Season with salt and pepper to taste.

6. Top with the remaining 2 toast slices to create 2 complete sandwiches.

7. Serve the vegan BLT sandwiches immediately.

Nutrition Information (per serving, 1 sandwich):
Calories: 320
Protein: 10g
Fat: 16g
Carbohydrates: 35g
Fiber: 6g
Vitamin A: 20% DV
Vitamin C: 15% DV

This Vegan BLT Sandwich is a delicious and satisfying plant-based take on the classic bacon, lettuce, and tomato sandwich. The vegan bacon provides a savory, smoky flavor, while the fresh tomatoes and crisp lettuce add a refreshing crunch.

12. Curried Cauliflower and Chickpea Salad

PreparationTime: 20 minutes

Cook Time: 20 minutes

Total Time: 40 minutes

Serves: 4

- 1 head of cauliflower, cut into florets
- 1 (15 oz) can chickpeas, drained and rinsed
- 2 tbsp olive oil
- 2 tsp curry powder
- 1/2 tsp ground cumin
- 1/4 tsp cayenne pepper (optional)
- Salt and pepper to taste
- 1/4 cup plain Greek yogurt (or vegan yogurt)
- 2 tbsp lemon juice
- 2 tbsp chopped fresh cilantro
- 2 tbsp chopped green onions
- 1/4 cup toasted slivered almonds

1. Preheat the oven to 400°F (200°C).

2. In a large bowl, toss the cauliflower florets and drained chickpeas with the olive oil, curry powder, cumin, and cayenne pepper (if using). Season with salt and pepper.

3. Spread the cauliflower and chickpea mixture on a baking sheet lined with parchment paper.

4. Roast in the preheated oven for 18-20 minutes, stirring halfway, until the cauliflower is tender and lightly browned.

5. Remove the roasted cauliflower and chickpeas from the oven and let them cool slightly.

6. In a large bowl, combine the roasted cauliflower and chickpeas with the Greek yogurt, lemon juice, chopped cilantro, and chopped green onions. Toss gently to coat.

7. Sprinkle the toasted slivered almonds over the top of the salad.

8. Serve the curried cauliflower and chickpea salad chilled or at room temperature.

Nutrition Information (per serving):
Calories: 220
Protein: 9g
Fat: 12g
Carbohydrates: 20g
Fiber: 7g
Vitamin A: 10% DV
Vitamin C: 70% DV

This Curried Cauliflower and Chickpea Salad is a flavorful and nutritious plant-based dish. The roasted cauliflower and chickpeas are tossed in a creamy curry-spiced dressing, making for a satisfying and delicious salad.

13. Creamy Tomato Basil Soup

PreparationTime: 15 minutes

Cook Time: 30 minutes

Total Time: 45 minutes

Serves: 4

- 2 tbsp olive oil
- 1 onion, diced
- 3 garlic cloves, minced
- 1 (28 oz) can crushed tomatoes
- 2 cups vegetable broth
- 1 cup unsweetened almond milk
- 1/4 cup raw cashews, soaked in water for at least 4 hours or overnight
- 1/4 cup fresh basil leaves, chopped
- 1 tsp dried oregano
- 1/4 tsp red pepper flakes (optional)
- Salt and pepper to taste
- Chopped fresh basil for garnish

Lunch

1. In a large pot or Dutch oven, heat the olive oil over medium heat. Add the diced onion and sauté for 5-7 minutes, until translucent.

2. Add the minced garlic and cook for an additional 1-2 minutes, until fragrant.

3. Stir in the crushed tomatoes, vegetable broth, and almond milk. Bring the mixture to a simmer.

4. Drain and rinse the soaked cashews, then add them to a high-speed blender. Blend until smooth and creamy.

5. Pour the blended cashew cream into the simmering tomato mixture. Stir in the chopped fresh basil, dried oregano, and red pepper flakes (if using).

6. Reduce the heat to low and let the soup simmer for 20-25 minutes, stirring occasionally, until slightly thickened.

7. Season with salt and pepper to taste.

8. Ladle the creamy tomato basil soup into bowls and garnish with additional chopped fresh basil. Serve hot, with crusty bread or grilled cheese sandwiches on the side.

Nutrition Information (per serving):
Calories: 220
Protein: 6g
Fat: 12g
Carbohydrates: 22g
Fiber: 5g
Vitamin A: 25% DV
Vitamin C: 20% DV

This Creamy Tomato Basil Soup is a comforting and flavorful plant-based dish. The addition of soaked cashews creates a rich and creamy texture, while the fresh basil and tomatoes provide a bright, aromatic flavor.

14. Falafel and Tabouli Wrap

PreparationTime: 30 minutes

Cook Time: 15 minutes

Total Time: 45 minutes

Serves: 4

For the Falafel:
- 1 (15 oz) can chickpeas, drained and rinsed
- 1/2 cup fresh parsley, chopped
- 1/4 cup fresh cilantro, chopped
- 2 garlic cloves, minced
- 1 tsp ground cumin
- 1/2 tsp ground coriander
- 1/4 tsp cayenne pepper
- 2 tbsp all-purpose flour
- Salt and pepper to taste
- 2 tbsp olive oil for frying

For the Tabouli:
- 1 cup bulgur wheat
- 1 cup chopped fresh parsley
- 1/2 cup chopped fresh mint
- 1 tomato, diced
- 1/2 cucumber, diced
- 2 tbsp lemon juice
- 2 tbsp olive oil
- Salt and pepper to taste

For the Wrap:
- 4 whole wheat tortillas or pita breads
- 1 cup shredded lettuce
- 1/2 cup hummus

Lunch

1. Make the falafel: In a food processor, combine the chickpeas, parsley, cilantro, garlic, cumin, coriander, and cayenne. Pulse until a coarse paste forms. Transfer to a bowl and stir in the flour, salt, and pepper.

2. Form the falafel mixture into small balls or patties, about 1-2 tablespoons each.

3. In a large skillet, heat the 2 tablespoons of olive oil over medium heat. Fry the falafel for 2-3 minutes per side, until golden brown. Drain on a paper towel-lined plate.

4. Make the tabouli: In a medium bowl, combine the bulgur wheat, chopped parsley, mint, diced tomato, and diced cucumber. Drizzle with lemon juice and olive oil, then season with salt and pepper. Toss to coat.

5. To assemble the wraps, spread a layer of hummus on each tortilla or pita. Top with shredded lettuce, a few falafel, and a scoop of the tabouli salad.

6. Fold the sides of the tortilla or pita over the filling and roll up tightly to create a wrap.

7. Serve the falafel and tabouli wraps immediately.

Nutrition Information (per serving):
Calories: 450
Protein: 14g
Fat: 18g
Carbohydrates: 58g
Fiber: 10g
Vitamin A: 30% DV
Vitamin C: 25% DV

This Falafel and Tabouli Wrap is a delicious and nutritious plant-based meal. The crispy falafel, fresh tabouli salad, and creamy hummus come together in a flavorful and satisfying wrap.

15. Vegan Greek Salad

PreparationTime: 20 minutes

Cook Time: 0 minutes

Total Time: 20 minutes

Serves: 4

- 1 cucumber, diced
- 1 pint cherry tomatoes, halved
- 1 red onion, thinly sliced
- 1 cup pitted kalamata olives, halved
- 1 cup crumbled vegan feta cheese (or regular feta if not vegan)
- 1/4 cup chopped fresh parsley
- 2 tbsp chopped fresh oregano
- 2 tbsp olive oil
- 2 tbsp red wine vinegar
- 1 tbsp lemon juice
- 1 garlic clove, minced
- 1/2 tsp Dijon mustard
- Salt and pepper to taste

Lunch

1. In a large salad bowl, combine the diced cucumber, halved cherry tomatoes, sliced red onion, halved kalamata olives, crumbled vegan feta cheese, chopped parsley, and chopped oregano.

2. In a small bowl, whisk together the olive oil, red wine vinegar, lemon juice, minced garlic, and Dijon mustard.

3. Pour the dressing over the salad and toss gently to coat.

4. Season the vegan Greek salad with salt and pepper to taste.

5. Serve immediately or refrigerate until ready to serve.

Nutrition Information (per serving):
Calories: 200
Protein: 6g
Fat: 15g
Carbohydrates: 14g
Fiber: 4g
Vitamin A: 20% DV
Vitamin C: 25% DV

This Vegan Greek Salad is a refreshing and flavorful plant-based dish. The combination of crisp vegetables, briny olives, and creamy vegan feta cheese, all tossed in a tangy vinaigrette, makes for a delicious and nutritious salad.

16. Sweet Potato and Lentil Stew

PreparationTime: 20 minutes

Cook Time: 40 minutes

Total Time: 1 hour

Serves: 4

- 1 tbsp olive oil
- 1 onion, diced
- 3 garlic cloves, minced
- 1 tbsp grated fresh ginger
- 1 tsp ground cumin
- 1 tsp ground coriander
- 1/2 tsp ground turmeric
- 1/4 tsp cayenne pepper (optional)
- 3 cups vegetable broth
- 1 cup dried red lentils, rinsed
- 2 medium sweet potatoes, peeled and cubed
- 1 (14 oz) can diced tomatoes
- 1 cup frozen peas
- Salt and pepper to taste
- Chopped fresh cilantro for garnish

Lunch

1. In a large pot or Dutch oven, heat the olive oil over medium heat. Add the diced onion and sauté for 5-7 minutes, until translucent.

2. Add the minced garlic, grated ginger, cumin, coriander, turmeric, and cayenne pepper (if using). Cook for 1-2 minutes, stirring constantly, until fragrant.

3. Pour in the vegetable broth and stir in the rinsed red lentils and cubed sweet potatoes.

4. Bring the stew to a boil, then reduce the heat to low, cover, and simmer for 30-35 minutes, or until the lentils and sweet potatoes are tender.

5. Stir in the diced tomatoes and frozen peas. Season with salt and pepper to taste.

6. Continue simmering the stew for an additional 5 minutes, or until the peas are heated through.

7. Ladle the sweet potato and lentil stew into bowls and garnish with chopped fresh cilantro.

8. Serve hot, with crusty bread or naan on the side.

Nutrition Information (per serving):
Calories: 350
Protein: 15g
Fat: 5g
Carbohydrates: 60g
Fiber: 12g
Vitamin A: 400% DV
Vitamin C: 25% DV

This Sweet Potato and Lentil Stew is a comforting and nutritious plant-based meal. The combination of sweet potatoes, lentils, and aromatic spices creates a flavorful and satisfying stew.

17. Vegan Chili with Cornbread

Preparation

- 1 tbsp olive oil
- 1 onion, diced
- 3 cloves garlic, minced
- 2 bell peppers, diced
- 2 cans (15 oz each) black beans, drained and rinsed
- 2 cans (15 oz each) kidney beans, drained and rinsed
- 1 can (28 oz) diced tomatoes
- 2 tbsp chili powder
- 1 tsp cumin
- 1 tsp oregano
- 1/2 tsp smoked paprika
- 1/4 tsp cayenne pepper (optional for heat)
- Salt and pepper to taste

Cornbread Ingredients:
- 1 cup cornmeal
- 1 cup all-purpose flour
- 2 tsp baking powder
- 1/2 tsp salt
- 1 cup unsweetened almond milk
- 1/4 cup maple syrup
- 2 tbsp olive oil

For the Chili:
1. In a large pot, heat the olive oil over medium heat. Add the onion and sauté for 5 minutes until translucent.
2. Add the garlic and bell peppers and sauté for 2-3 more minutes.
3. Stir in the black beans, kidney beans, diced tomatoes, chili powder, cumin, oregano, smoked paprika and cayenne (if using). Season with salt and pepper.
4. Bring to a simmer and let cook for 20-25 minutes, stirring occasionally, until thickened.

For the Cornbread:
1. Preheat oven to 400°F. Grease an 8-inch square baking pan.
2. In a medium bowl, whisk together the cornmeal, flour, baking powder and salt.
3. In a separate bowl, whisk together the almond milk, maple syrup and olive oil.
4. Pour the wet ingredients into the dry ingredients and stir just until combined (do not overmix).
5. Pour the cornbread batter into the prepared pan and bake for 18-22 minutes, until a toothpick inserted in the center comes out clean.

Serve the vegan chili warm, with slices of the cornbread on the side. Enjoy!

Lunch

18. Kale and Quinoa Salad with Lemon Tahini Dressing

PreparationTime: 20 minutes

Cook Time: 15 minutes

Total Time: 35 minutes

Serves: 4

For the Salad:
- 1 cup uncooked quinoa, rinsed
- 2 cups vegetable broth
- 4 cups chopped kale, stems removed
- 1 cup diced cucumber
- 1/2 cup diced red bell pepper
- 1/4 cup chopped fresh parsley
- 2 tbsp toasted pumpkin seeds

For the Lemon Tahini Dressing:
- 1/4 cup tahini
- 2 tbsp lemon juice
- 1 tbsp maple syrup
- 1 garlic clove, minced
- 2 tbsp water
- Salt and pepper to taste

Lunch

1. In a medium saucepan, combine the rinsed quinoa and vegetable broth. Bring to a boil, then reduce heat to low, cover, and simmer for 15 minutes, or until the quinoa is cooked and the liquid is absorbed. Fluff with a fork and set aside to cool.

2. In a large salad bowl, combine the chopped kale, diced cucumber, diced red bell pepper, and chopped parsley.

3. In a small bowl, whisk together the tahini, lemon juice, maple syrup, minced garlic, and water. Season with salt and pepper to taste.

4. Add the cooked and cooled quinoa to the salad bowl. Drizzle the lemon tahini dressing over the salad and toss to coat everything evenly.

5. Sprinkle the toasted pumpkin seeds over the top of the salad.

6. Serve the kale and quinoa salad immediately, or refrigerate until ready to serve.

Nutrition Information (per serving):
Calories: 320
Protein: 12g
Fat: 14g
Carbohydrates: 38g
Fiber: 7g
Vitamin A: 120% DV
Vitamin C: 80% DV

This Kale and Quinoa Salad with Lemon Tahini Dressing is a nutritious and flavorful plant-based meal. The combination of nutrient-dense kale, protein-rich quinoa, and the creamy tahini dressing makes for a satisfying and delicious salad.

19. Vegan Ramen with Tofu

Preparation

- 8 oz ramen noodles
- 4 cups vegetable broth
- 2 tbsp soy sauce or tamari
- 1 tbsp rice vinegar
- 1 tsp sesame oil
- 1 tsp grated ginger
- 2 cloves garlic, minced
- 1/4 tsp red pepper flakes (optional)
- 8 oz firm or extra-firm tofu, cubed
- 2 cups shredded cabbage or spinach
- 1 carrot, julienned or shredded
- 2 green onions, sliced
- Sesame seeds for garnish

1. Bring a large pot of water to a boil. Cook the ramen noodles according to package Directions, then drain and set aside.

2. In a separate pot, combine the vegetable broth, soy sauce, rice vinegar, sesame oil, ginger, garlic and red pepper flakes (if using). Bring to a simmer over medium heat.

3. Add the cubed tofu to the simmering broth and cook for 5-7 minutes, until heated through.

4. Add the cooked ramen noodles, shredded cabbage/spinach and julienned carrot to the broth. Cook for 2-3 minutes, until the vegetables are slightly wilted.

5. Remove from heat and ladle the ramen into bowls. Top each serving with sliced green onions and a sprinkle of sesame seeds.

Serve the vegan ramen hot, with extra soy sauce or chili oil on the side if desired.

Enjoy!

Lunch

20. Roasted Beet and Citrus Salad

Preparation

- 3 medium beets, peeled and cut into 1-inch cubes
- 2 tbsp olive oil
- Salt and pepper to taste
- 1 orange, peeled and segmented
- 1 grapefruit, peeled and segmented
- 1 avocado, diced
- 2 cups mixed greens
- 2 tbsp crumbled feta cheese (optional)
- 2 tbsp toasted walnuts or pecans

Dressing:
- 2 tbsp olive oil
- 1 tbsp orange juice
- 1 tbsp grapefruit juice
- 1 tbsp white wine vinegar
- 1 tsp Dijon mustard
- 1 tsp honey
- Salt and pepper to taste

Lunch

1. Preheat oven to 400°F. Toss the cubed beets with 2 tbsp olive oil and season with salt and pepper. Spread on a baking sheet.

2. Roast the beets for 25-30 minutes, stirring halfway, until tender and caramelized. Let cool slightly.

3. In a large bowl, combine the roasted beets, orange segments, grapefruit segments, avocado and mixed greens.

4. In a small bowl, whisk together the dressing ingredients - olive oil, orange juice, grapefruit juice, vinegar, mustard, honey, salt and pepper.

5. Drizzle the dressing over the salad and gently toss to coat.

6. Top the salad with crumbled feta cheese (if using) and toasted nuts.

Serve the roasted beet and citrus salad chilled or at room temperature. Enjoy!

1. Vegan Lentil Bolognese

Preparation

- 1 cup dry brown or green lentils, rinsed
- 4 cups vegetable broth
- 1 tbsp olive oil
- 1 onion, diced
- 3 cloves garlic, minced
- 1 carrot, peeled and diced
- 1 celery stalk, diced
- 1 (28 oz) can diced tomatoes
- 2 tbsp tomato paste
- 1 tsp dried oregano
- 1 tsp dried basil
- 1/2 tsp red pepper flakes (optional)
- Salt and pepper to taste
- Cooked pasta, for serving

Dinner

1. In a medium saucepan, combine the lentils and vegetable broth. Bring to a boil, then reduce heat and simmer for 20-25 minutes, until lentils are tender. Drain any excess liquid and set aside.

2. In a large skillet, heat the olive oil over medium heat. Add the onion and sauté for 5 minutes until translucent.

3. Add the garlic, carrot and celery. Sauté for 3-4 minutes more, until vegetables are softened.

4. Stir in the diced tomatoes, tomato paste, oregano, basil and red pepper flakes (if using). Season with salt and pepper.

5. Add the cooked lentils to the tomato sauce mixture and stir to combine. Simmer for 10-15 minutes, allowing the flavors to meld.

6. Serve the vegan lentil bolognese over cooked pasta of your choice. Top with fresh basil, vegan parmesan or other desired toppings.

Enjoy this hearty, plant-based take on a classic Italian dish!

2. Stuffed Acorn Squash with Wild Rice

PreparationTime: 15 minutes

Cook Time: 50 minutes

Total Time: 1 hour 5 minutes

Serves: 4

- 2 acorn squash, halved and seeded
- 1 cup cooked wild rice
- 1/2 cup diced onion
- 1/2 cup diced celery
- 1/2 cup diced mushrooms
- 2 cloves garlic, minced
- 1 tsp dried thyme
- 1/4 cup dried cranberries
- 1/4 cup toasted pecans or walnuts
- Salt and pepper to taste
- 2 tbsp olive oil

Dinner

1. Preheat oven to 400°F. Place the acorn squash halves cut-side up on a baking sheet. Brush the insides with 1 tbsp of the olive oil and season with salt and pepper.

2. Roast the squash for 30-40 minutes, until tender when pierced with a fork.

3. In a skillet, heat the remaining 1 tbsp olive oil over medium heat. Add the onion, celery, mushrooms and garlic. Sauté for 5-7 minutes until vegetables are softened.

4. Remove from heat and stir in the cooked wild rice, thyme, cranberries and toasted nuts. Season with salt and pepper to taste.

5. Scoop the wild rice stuffing into the roasted acorn squash halves, dividing it evenly.

6. Return the stuffed squash to the oven and bake for an additional 10-15 minutes, until heated through.

7. Serve the stuffed acorn squash warm.

Enjoy!

3. Chickpea and Spinach Curry

PreparationTime: 15 minutes

Cook Time: 30 minutes

Total Time: 45 minutes

Serves: 4

- 1 tablespoon olive oil
- 1 onion, diced
- 3 cloves garlic, minced
- 1 tablespoon grated ginger
- 1 tablespoon garam masala
- 1 teaspoon ground cumin
- 1 teaspoon ground coriander
- 1/2 teaspoon cayenne pepper (or to taste)
- 1 (15 oz) can chickpeas, drained and rinsed
- 1 (14 oz) can diced tomatoes
- 1 cup vegetable broth
- 5 oz fresh spinach, roughly chopped
- Salt and pepper to taste
- Chopped cilantro for garnish

1. In a large skillet or pot, heat the olive oil over medium heat. Add the onion and sauté for 5 minutes until translucent.

2. Add the garlic and ginger and cook for 1 minute, until fragrant.

3. Stir in the garam masala, cumin, coriander, and cayenne. Cook for 2 minutes to toast the spices.

4. Add the chickpeas, diced tomatoes, and vegetable broth. Bring to a simmer and cook for 20 minutes, stirring occasionally, until the sauce has thickened.

5. Stir in the chopped spinach and cook for 2-3 minutes until the spinach is wilted.

6. Season with salt and pepper to taste.

7. Serve the chickpea and spinach curry over basmati rice or with naan bread. Garnish with chopped cilantro.

Enjoy this flavorful and nutritious chickpea and spinach curry! The combination of spices, chickpeas, and fresh spinach makes for a delicious and satisfying vegetarian meal.

Dinner

4. Eggplant Parmesan

PreparationTime: 30 minutes
Cook Time: 45 minutes
Total Time: 1 hour 15 minutes
Serves: 4-6

- 2 medium eggplants, sliced into 1/2-inch thick rounds
- 1 cup all-purpose flour
- 2 eggs, beaten
- 2 cups panko breadcrumbs
- 1/2 cup grated Parmesan cheese
- 1 tsp dried oregano
- 1 tsp dried basil
- Salt and pepper to taste
- 2 cups marinara sauce
- 2 cups shredded mozzarella cheese

Dinner

1. Preheat oven to 375°F. Line a baking sheet with parchment paper.

2. Dredge the eggplant slices in flour, dip in the beaten eggs, and then coat in the panko breadcrumb mixture mixed with Parmesan, oregano, basil, salt, and pepper.

3. Arrange the breaded eggplant slices in a single layer on the prepared baking sheet.

4. Bake for 20-25 minutes, flipping halfway, until the eggplant is golden brown and crispy.

5. Spread 1 cup of the marinara sauce in the bottom of a 9x13 inch baking dish.

6. Arrange the baked eggplant slices in a single layer on top of the sauce. Top with the remaining 1 cup of marinara sauce and the shredded mozzarella cheese.

7. Bake for an additional 20-25 minutes, until the cheese is melted and bubbly.

8. Let stand for 5 minutes before serving.

Serve the eggplant parmesan hot, garnished with fresh basil if desired. Enjoy this classic Italian-inspired dish!

5. Vegan Mushroom Stroganoff

PreparationTime: 20 minutes

Cook Time: 30 minutes

Total Time: 50 minutes

Serves: 4

- 8 oz cremini mushrooms, sliced
- 8 oz shiitake mushrooms, sliced
- 1 onion, diced
- 3 garlic cloves, minced
- 2 tbsp olive oil
- 2 tbsp all-purpose flour
- 1 cup vegetable broth
- 1 cup unsweetened almond milk
- 2 tsp Dijon mustard
- 2 tsp soy sauce
- 1 tsp dried thyme
- Salt and pepper to taste
- 8 oz egg-free egg noodles
- Chopped parsley for garnish

1. Bring a large pot of salted water to a boil for the egg noodles.

2. In a large skillet, heat the olive oil over medium-high heat. Add the mushrooms, onion, and garlic. Sauté for 5-7 minutes until the mushrooms are browned and the onions are translucent.

3. Sprinkle the flour over the mushroom mixture and stir to coat. Cook for 2 minutes.

4. Gradually whisk in the vegetable broth and almond milk. Bring to a simmer and cook for 5-7 minutes, until the sauce has thickened.

5. Stir in the Dijon mustard, soy sauce, and thyme. Season with salt and pepper to taste.

6. Meanwhile, cook the egg noodles according to package Directions. Drain and set aside.

7. Add the cooked noodles to the mushroom stroganoff and toss to combine.

8. Serve the vegan mushroom stroganoff hot, garnished with chopped parsley.

Enjoy this rich and creamy vegan mushroom stroganoff! The combination of savory mushrooms, tangy Dijon, and tender noodles makes for a delicious plant-based meal.

Dinner

6. Sweet Potato and Black Bean Enchiladas

PreparationTime: 30 minutes

Cook Time: 30 minutes

Total Time: 1 hour

Serves: 4-6

- 2 medium sweet potatoes, peeled and diced
- 1 tbsp olive oil
- 1 onion, diced
- 3 garlic cloves, minced
- 1 (15 oz) can black beans, drained and rinsed
- 1 tsp ground cumin
- 1 tsp chili powder
- Salt and pepper to taste
- 12 corn tortillas
- 2 cups enchilada sauce
- 1 cup shredded vegan cheddar cheese

1. Preheat oven to 375°F. Grease a 9x13 inch baking dish.

2. In a large skillet, heat the olive oil over medium heat. Add the diced sweet potatoes and sauté for 8-10 minutes, until tender.

3. Add the onion and garlic to the skillet and cook for 2-3 minutes until fragrant.

4. Stir in the black beans, cumin, chili powder, salt, and pepper. Cook for 2-3 minutes more.

5. Spread 1/2 cup of the enchilada sauce in the bottom of the prepared baking dish.

6. Spoon about 1/4 cup of the sweet potato and black bean mixture onto each corn tortilla. Roll up the tortillas and place seam-side down in the baking dish.

7. Pour the remaining 1 1/2 cups of enchilada sauce over the rolled enchiladas. Sprinkle the shredded vegan cheese on top.

8. Bake for 20-25 minutes, until the cheese is melted and the enchiladas are heated through.

9. Let stand for 5 minutes before serving.

Serve the sweet potato and black bean enchiladas warm, garnished with chopped cilantro if desired. Enjoy this flavorful and satisfying vegetarian Mexican dish!

Dinner

7. Cauliflower and Chickpea Tacos

PreparationTime: 20 minutes

Cook Time: 30 minutes

Total Time: 50 minutes

Serves: 4-6

- 1 head of cauliflower, cut into florets
- 1 (15 oz) can chickpeas, drained and rinsed
- 2 tbsp olive oil
- 1 tsp chili powder
- 1 tsp cumin
- 1/2 tsp garlic powder
- Salt and pepper to taste
- 12-16 small corn tortillas
- 1 cup shredded red cabbage
- 1 avocado, sliced
- 1/4 cup chopped cilantro
- Lime wedges for serving

For the Taco Sauce:
- 1/2 cup plain Greek yogurt or vegan sour cream
- 2 tbsp lime juice
- 1 tsp Dijon mustard
- 1 tsp maple syrup
- Salt and pepper to taste

Dinner

1. Preheat oven to 400°F. Line a baking sheet with parchment paper.

2. In a large bowl, toss the cauliflower florets and chickpeas with the olive oil, chili powder, cumin, garlic powder, salt, and pepper. Spread in a single layer on the prepared baking sheet.

3. Roast for 25-30 minutes, stirring halfway, until the cauliflower is tender and lightly browned.

4. Meanwhile, make the taco sauce by whisking together the yogurt/sour cream, lime juice, Dijon, maple syrup, salt, and pepper.

5. Warm the corn tortillas according to package Directions.

6. To assemble the tacos, place some of the roasted cauliflower and chickpea mixture into each tortilla. Top with shredded cabbage, avocado slices, and a drizzle of the taco sauce.

7. Garnish with chopped cilantro and serve with lime wedges.

Enjoy these flavorful and nutritious cauliflower and chickpea tacos! The combination of roasted veggies, creamy sauce, and fresh toppings makes for a delicious plant-based meal.

8. Vegan Shepherd's Pie

PreparationTime: 30 minutes

Cook Time: 45 minutes

Total Time: 1 hour 15 minutes

Serves: 4-6

For the Mashed Potato Topping:
- 2 lbs russet potatoes, peeled and cut into 1-inch chunks
- 1/4 cup unsweetened almond milk
- 2 tbsp vegan butter
- Salt and pepper to taste

For the Filling:
- 1 tbsp olive oil
- 1 onion, diced
- 3 carrots, peeled and diced
- 3 celery stalks, diced
- 3 garlic cloves, minced
- 1 tsp dried thyme
- 1 tsp dried rosemary
- 1 (15 oz) can diced tomatoes
- 1 (15 oz) can kidney beans, drained and rinsed
- 1 (15 oz) can green peas, drained
- 2 cups vegetable broth
- 2 tbsp tomato paste
- 2 tbsp all-purpose flour
- Salt and pepper to taste

Dinner

1. Preheat oven to 375°F.

2. Make the mashed potato topping: Place the potato chunks in a pot and cover with water. Bring to a boil and cook until tender, about 15 minutes. Drain and return to the pot. Mash with the almond milk and vegan butter. Season with salt and pepper.

3. Make the filling: In a large skillet, heat the olive oil over medium heat. Add the onion, carrots, celery and garlic. Cook for 5-7 minutes until softened.

4. Stir in the thyme, rosemary, diced tomatoes, kidney beans, peas, vegetable broth, tomato paste and flour. Bring to a simmer and cook for 10 minutes, until thickened.

5. Transfer the vegetable mixture to a 9x13 inch baking dish. Spread the mashed potatoes evenly over the top.

6. Bake for 25-30 minutes, until the potatoes are lightly browned on top.

7. Let stand for 5 minutes before serving.

Enjoy this hearty and comforting vegan shepherd's pie! The mashed potato topping is the perfect complement to the savory vegetable filling.

9. Spaghetti with Vegan Meatballs

PreparationTime: 30 minutes

Cook Time: 45 minutes

Total Time: 1 hour 15 minutes

Serves: 4-6

For the Vegan Meatballs:
- 1 cup cooked brown rice
- 1 (15 oz) can chickpeas, drained and rinsed
- 1/2 cup panko breadcrumbs
- 1/4 cup grated vegan parmesan cheese
- 2 tbsp ground flaxseed
- 2 garlic cloves, minced
- 1 tsp dried oregano
- 1/2 tsp dried basil
- 1/4 tsp red pepper flakes
- Salt and pepper to taste

For the Spaghetti:
- 12 oz spaghetti
- 1 tbsp olive oil
- 1 onion, diced
- 3 garlic cloves, minced
- 1 (28 oz) can crushed tomatoes
- 2 tbsp tomato paste
- 1 tsp dried oregano
- 1/2 tsp dried basil
- Salt and pepper to taste
- Chopped fresh basil for garnish

Dinner

1. Preheat oven to 375°F. Line a baking sheet with parchment paper.

2. Make the vegan meatballs: In a food processor, combine the cooked rice, chickpeas, breadcrumbs, vegan parmesan, flaxseed, garlic, oregano, basil, red pepper flakes, salt, and pepper. Pulse until the mixture comes together but is still slightly chunky.

3. Scoop the mixture by heaping tablespoons and roll into 1-inch meatballs. Place on the prepared baking sheet.

4. Bake the meatballs for 20-25 minutes, turning halfway, until lightly browned.

5. Meanwhile, bring a large pot of salted water to a boil. Cook the spaghetti according to package Directions until al dente. Drain and set aside.

6. In a large skillet, heat the olive oil over medium heat. Add the onion and garlic and cook for 2-3 minutes until fragrant.

7. Stir in the crushed tomatoes, tomato paste, oregano, basil, salt, and pepper. Simmer for 10-15 minutes, until the sauce has thickened.

8. Add the cooked spaghetti and vegan meatballs to the sauce and toss to coat.

9. Serve the spaghetti and meatballs hot, garnished with chopped fresh basil.

Enjoy this delicious and satisfying vegan spaghetti and meatball dish! The homemade vegan meatballs are the perfect complement to the flavorful tomato sauce.

10. Moroccan Vegetable Tagine

PreparationTime: 30 minutes

Cook Time: 45 minutes

Total Time: 1 hour 15 minutes

Serves: 4-6

- 2 tbsp olive oil
- 1 onion, diced
- 3 garlic cloves, minced
- 1 tsp ground cumin
- 1 tsp ground coriander
- 1 tsp paprika
- 1/2 tsp ground cinnamon
- 1/4 tsp cayenne pepper (or to taste)
- 1 (15 oz) can diced tomatoes
- 1 cup vegetable broth
- 1 lb sweet potatoes, peeled and cubed
- 1 lb butternut squash, peeled and cubed
- 1 (15 oz) can chickpeas, drained and rinsed
- 1 cup green beans, trimmed and cut into 1-inch pieces
- 1 cup cauliflower florets
- 1/4 cup chopped cilantro
- 1/4 cup chopped parsley
- Salt and pepper to taste
- Cooked couscous or quinoa, for serving

Dinner

1. In a large pot or Dutch oven, heat the olive oil over medium heat. Add the onion and sauté for 5 minutes until translucent.

2. Add the garlic, cumin, coriander, paprika, cinnamon, and cayenne. Cook for 1 minute, until fragrant.

3. Stir in the diced tomatoes, vegetable broth, sweet potatoes, butternut squash, chickpeas, green beans, and cauliflower. Season with salt and pepper.

4. Bring the mixture to a simmer, then reduce heat to medium-low. Cover and cook for 30-35 minutes, until the vegetables are tender.

5. Remove from heat and stir in the chopped cilantro and parsley.

6. Serve the Moroccan vegetable tagine warm, over cooked couscous or quinoa.

Enjoy this flavorful and nourishing Moroccan-inspired vegetable tagine! The blend of aromatic spices, roasted vegetables, and chickpeas makes for a delicious and satisfying plant-based meal.

11. Vegan Alfredo Pasta

PreparationTime: 20 minutes

Cook Time: 20 minutes

Total Time: 40 minutes

Serves: 4

- 12 oz fettuccine pasta
- 1 cup raw cashews, soaked in water for at least 4 hours or overnight
- 1 cup unsweetened almond milk
- 2 garlic cloves, minced
- 2 tbsp nutritional yeast
- 1 tsp lemon juice
- 1/2 tsp salt
- 1/4 tsp ground black pepper
- Chopped parsley for garnish

Dinner

1. Bring a large pot of salted water to a boil. Cook the fettuccine according to package Directions until al dente. Drain and set aside.

2. Drain and rinse the soaked cashews. Add them to a high-speed blender along with the almond milk, garlic, nutritional yeast, lemon juice, salt, and pepper. Blend until smooth and creamy.

3. In a large skillet, heat the cashew alfredo sauce over medium heat, stirring occasionally, until warmed through and slightly thickened, about 5 minutes.

4. Add the cooked fettuccine to the sauce and toss to coat the noodles evenly.

5. Serve the vegan alfredo pasta hot, garnished with chopped parsley.

Optional add-ins:
- Sautéed mushrooms or spinach
- Grilled or roasted vegetables
- Crispy tofu or tempeh

This creamy vegan alfredo pasta is a delicious and dairy-free twist on the classic dish. The cashew-based sauce provides a rich and indulgent texture without any animal products. Enjoy this comforting plant-based meal!

12. Roasted Vegetable and Quinoa Stuffed Peppers

PreparationTime: 30 minutes

Cook Time: 45 minutes

Total Time: 1 hour 15 minutes

Serves: 4-6

- 6 bell peppers, halved lengthwise and seeds removed
- 1 cup uncooked quinoa, rinsed
- 2 cups vegetable broth
- 1 tbsp olive oil
- 1 onion, diced
- 3 garlic cloves, minced
- 1 cup diced zucchini
- 1 cup diced eggplant
- 1 cup diced mushrooms
- 1 tsp dried oregano
- 1 tsp dried basil
- Salt and pepper to taste
- 1 cup shredded vegan mozzarella cheese (optional)
- Chopped parsley for garnish

1. Preheat oven to 375°F. Place the bell pepper halves cut-side up in a baking dish. Set aside.

2. In a medium saucepan, combine the quinoa and vegetable broth. Bring to a boil, then reduce heat to low, cover, and simmer for 15-20 minutes until the quinoa is cooked and liquid is absorbed. Fluff with a fork and set aside.

3. In a large skillet, heat the olive oil over medium heat. Add the onion and sauté for 3-4 minutes until translucent.

4. Add the garlic, zucchini, eggplant, and mushrooms. Cook for 5-7 minutes, stirring occasionally, until the vegetables are tender.

5. Stir the cooked quinoa, oregano, basil, salt, and pepper into the vegetable mixture until well combined.

6. Spoon the quinoa and vegetable filling into the bell pepper halves, packing it in tightly.

7. Cover the baking dish with foil and bake for 30 minutes. Remove the foil and bake for an additional 10-15 minutes, until the peppers are tender.

8. If using, sprinkle the shredded vegan cheese over the top of the stuffed peppers during the last 5 minutes of baking.

9. Serve the roasted vegetable and quinoa stuffed peppers warm, garnished with chopped parsley.

Enjoy this healthy and flavorful plant-based stuffed pepper dish! The combination of roasted veggies and protein-packed quinoa makes for a satisfying and nutritious meal.

Dinner

13. Mushroom and Lentil Loaf

PreparationTime: 30 minutes

Cook Time: 1 hour

Total Time: 1 hour 30 minutes

Serves: 6-8

- 1 cup brown or green lentils, rinsed
- 3 cups vegetable broth
- 1 tbsp olive oil
- 1 onion, diced
- 8 oz cremini mushrooms, finely chopped
- 3 garlic cloves, minced
- 1 tsp dried thyme
- 1 tsp dried rosemary
- 1 cup rolled oats
- 1/2 cup breadcrumbs
- 2 tbsp ground flaxseed
- 2 tbsp soy sauce or tamari
- 1 tsp Dijon mustard
- Salt and pepper to taste

For the Glaze:
- 1/4 cup ketchup
- 2 tbsp maple syrup
- 1 tbsp apple cider vinegar

Dinner

1. Preheat oven to 375°F. Grease a 9x5 inch loaf pan.

2. In a medium saucepan, combine the lentils and vegetable broth. Bring to a boil, then reduce heat and simmer for 20-25 minutes, until the lentils are tender. Drain any excess liquid and set aside.

3. In a large skillet, heat the olive oil over medium heat. Add the onion and sauté for 5 minutes until translucent.

4. Add the chopped mushrooms and garlic. Cook for 5-7 minutes, until the mushrooms are softened.

5. Transfer the cooked lentils and mushroom mixture to a large bowl. Stir in the thyme, rosemary, rolled oats, breadcrumbs, flaxseed, soy sauce, and Dijon. Season with salt and pepper.

6. Press the lentil mixture firmly into the prepared loaf pan.

7. In a small bowl, whisk together the ingredients for the glaze. Spread the glaze evenly over the top of the loaf.

8. Bake for 45-55 minutes, until the top is browned and the loaf is firm.

9. Let the loaf cool in the pan for 10 minutes before slicing and serving.

Serve the mushroom and lentil loaf warm, with your choice of sides. Enjoy this hearty and flavorful plant-based main dish!

14. Vegan Pad Thai

PreparationTime: 20 minutes

Cook Time: 20 minutes

Total Time: 40 minutes

Serves: 4

- 8 oz rice noodles
- 2 tbsp vegetable oil
- 1 block extra-firm tofu, pressed and cubed
- 3 cloves garlic, minced
- 1 cup bean sprouts
- 1 cup shredded carrots
- 1/2 cup chopped green onions
- 1/4 cup chopped roasted peanuts
- 2 tbsp chopped cilantro

For the Sauce:
- 3 tbsp tamarind paste
- 2 tbsp soy sauce or tamari
- 2 tbsp brown sugar
- 1 tbsp rice vinegar
- 1 tsp chili garlic sauce (or to taste)
- 1 tsp lime juice
- 1 tsp sesame oil

Dinner

1. Soak the rice noodles in hot water for 15-20 minutes, until softened. Drain and set aside.

2. In a small bowl, whisk together all the sauce ingredients. Set aside.

3. In a large skillet or wok, heat the vegetable oil over medium-high heat. Add the cubed tofu and cook for 3-4 minutes per side, until lightly browned. Transfer to a plate.

4. Add the garlic to the skillet and cook for 1 minute until fragrant.

5. Add the softened rice noodles and sauce to the skillet. Toss everything together for 2-3 minutes, until the noodles are evenly coated and heated through.

6. Stir in the cooked tofu, bean sprouts, carrots, and green onions. Toss to combine.

7. Remove from heat and garnish the vegan pad thai with chopped peanuts and cilantro.

8. Serve immediately while hot.

Enjoy this flavorful and authentic-tasting vegan pad thai! The combination of chewy rice noodles, crispy tofu, and fresh veggies in the sweet and tangy sauce makes for a delicious plant-based meal.

15. Tofu Stir-Fry with Broccoli and Cashews

PreparationTime: 20 minutes

Cook Time: 20 minutes

Total Time: 40 minutes

Serves: 4

- 1 block extra-firm tofu, pressed and cubed
- 2 tbsp vegetable oil, divided
- 3 cups broccoli florets
- 1 red bell pepper, sliced
- 3 cloves garlic, minced
- 1 tbsp grated ginger
- 1/2 cup unsalted cashews
- 2 tbsp soy sauce or tamari
- 1 tbsp rice vinegar
- 1 tsp sesame oil
- 1 tsp maple syrup
- Salt and pepper to taste
- Cooked rice, for serving

Dinner

1. In a large skillet or wok, heat 1 tbsp of the vegetable oil over medium-high heat. Add the cubed tofu and cook for 5-7 minutes, turning occasionally, until lightly browned on all sides. Transfer the tofu to a plate.

2. In the same skillet, heat the remaining 1 tbsp of oil. Add the broccoli florets and bell pepper slices. Stir-fry for 5-7 minutes until the vegetables are tender-crisp.

3. Add the garlic and ginger to the skillet. Cook for 1 minute until fragrant.

4. Return the cooked tofu to the skillet. Add the cashews, soy sauce, rice vinegar, sesame oil, and maple syrup. Toss everything together and cook for 2-3 minutes, until heated through.

5. Season the stir-fry with salt and pepper to taste.

6. Serve the tofu and vegetable stir-fry immediately over cooked rice.

Garnish with additional chopped cashews or green onions if desired.

This tofu stir-fry with broccoli and cashews is a quick, flavorful, and nutritious plant-based meal. The combination of crispy tofu, fresh veggies, and crunchy cashews in a savory sauce makes for a delicious and satisfying dish.

16. Vegan Lasagna with Spinach and Tofu Ricotta

PreparationTime: 45 minutes

Cook Time: 1 hour

Total Time: 1 hour 45 minutes

Serves: 6-8

For the Tofu Ricotta:
- 1 block (14 oz) extra-firm tofu, drained and crumbled
- 1/4 cup raw cashews, soaked in water for 4 hours or overnight
- 2 tbsp lemon juice
- 2 tbsp nutritional yeast
- 1 tsp dried oregano
- 1/2 tsp garlic powder
- 1/4 tsp salt

For the Lasagna:
- 9 lasagna noodles
- 1 tbsp olive oil
- 1 onion, diced
- 3 garlic cloves, minced
- 1 (28 oz) can crushed tomatoes
- 2 tbsp tomato paste
- 1 tsp dried basil
- 1 tsp dried oregano
- Salt and pepper to taste
- 5 oz baby spinach
- 1 cup shredded vegan mozzarella cheese

Dinner

1. Make the tofu ricotta: Drain and crumble the tofu into a food processor. Add the soaked cashews, lemon juice, nutritional yeast, oregano, garlic powder, and salt. Pulse until a ricotta-like texture forms. Set aside.

2. Preheat oven to 375°F. Bring a large pot of salted water to a boil. Cook the lasagna noodles according to package Directions until al dente. Drain and set aside.

3. In a large skillet, heat the olive oil over medium heat. Add the onion and sauté for 5 minutes until translucent.

4. Add the garlic and cook for 1 minute until fragrant. Stir in the crushed tomatoes, tomato paste, basil, oregano, salt, and pepper. Simmer for 10 minutes.

5. Spread 1/2 cup of the tomato sauce in the bottom of a 9x13 inch baking dish.

6. Layer 3 lasagna noodles over the sauce. Spread half of the tofu ricotta over the noodles, then top with half of the spinach.

7. Repeat the layers of noodles, tofu ricotta, and spinach. Top with the remaining 3 noodles and the remaining tomato sauce.

8. Sprinkle the shredded vegan mozzarella cheese over the top.

9. Cover the dish with foil and bake for 45 minutes. Remove the foil and bake for an additional 15 minutes, until the cheese is melted and bubbly.

10. Let the lasagna stand for 10 minutes before slicing and serving.

17. Grilled Portobello Mushrooms with Balsamic Glaze

PreparationTime: 15 minutes

Cook Time: 20 minutes

Total Time: 35 minutes

Serves: 4

- 4 large portobello mushrooms, stems removed
- 2 tbsp olive oil
- 1/4 cup balsamic vinegar
- 2 tbsp maple syrup
- 2 garlic cloves, minced
- 1 tsp dried thyme
- Salt and pepper to taste
- Chopped parsley for garnish

Dinner

1. Preheat grill or grill pan to medium-high heat.

2. In a shallow baking dish, whisk together the olive oil, balsamic vinegar, maple syrup, garlic, and thyme. Season with salt and pepper.

3. Add the portobello mushrooms to the balsamic mixture, turning to coat both sides.

4. Grill the mushrooms for 5-7 minutes per side, basting with the remaining balsamic mixture, until tender and lightly charred.

5. Transfer the grilled portobello mushrooms to a serving platter.

6. In a small saucepan, bring the remaining balsamic mixture to a simmer over medium heat. Cook for 2-3 minutes, stirring frequently, until thickened into a glaze.

7. Drizzle the balsamic glaze over the grilled portobello mushrooms.

8. Garnish with chopped parsley before serving.

Serve the grilled portobello mushrooms warm, as a main dish or appetizer. The balsamic glaze adds a sweet and tangy flavor that complements the meaty texture of the mushrooms.

This simple yet flavorful recipe is a great option for a plant-based grilling or summer meal. Enjoy!

18. Vegan Jambalaya

PreparationTime: 20 minutes

Cook Time: 40 minutes

Total Time: 1 hour

Serves: 4-6

- 1 cup uncooked long-grain white rice
- 2 cups vegetable broth
- 1 tbsp olive oil
- 1 onion, diced
- 1 green bell pepper, diced
- 3 celery stalks, diced
- 3 garlic cloves, minced
- 1 tsp smoked paprika
- 1 tsp dried thyme
- 1 tsp dried oregano
- 1/2 tsp cayenne pepper (or to taste)
- 1 (14 oz) can diced tomatoes
- 1 (15 oz) can kidney beans, drained and rinsed
- 1 (15 oz) can chickpeas, drained and rinsed
- 1 cup chopped vegan sausage or seitan (optional)
- Salt and pepper to taste
- Chopped parsley for garnish

1. In a medium saucepan, combine the rice and vegetable broth. Bring to a boil, then reduce heat, cover, and simmer for 20 minutes until the rice is tender. Fluff with a fork and set aside.

2. In a large skillet or Dutch oven, heat the olive oil over medium heat. Add the onion, bell pepper, and celery. Sauté for 5-7 minutes until the vegetables are softened.

3. Stir in the garlic, smoked paprika, thyme, oregano, and cayenne. Cook for 1 minute until fragrant.

4. Add the diced tomatoes, kidney beans, chickpeas, and vegan sausage (if using). Simmer for 15-20 minutes, stirring occasionally, until the flavors have melded.

5. Stir the cooked rice into the jambalaya mixture until well combined.

6. Season with salt and pepper to taste.

7. Serve the vegan jambalaya hot, garnished with chopped parsley.

This plant-based jambalaya is packed with flavor and protein-rich ingredients like beans and rice. It's a delicious and satisfying one-pot meal. Adjust the spice level to your preference.

Dinner

19. Stuffed Zucchini Boats

PreparationTime: 20 minutes

Cook Time: 30 minutes

Total Time: 50 minutes

Serves: 4

- 4 medium zucchini, halved lengthwise
- 1 tbsp olive oil
- 1 onion, diced
- 2 garlic cloves, minced
- 8 oz cremini mushrooms, diced
- 1 (15 oz) can diced tomatoes
- 1 cup cooked quinoa
- 1/2 cup shredded vegan mozzarella cheese
- 2 tbsp chopped fresh basil
- Salt and pepper to taste

Dinner

1. Preheat oven to 375°F. Scoop out the flesh from the zucchini halves, leaving about 1/4 inch of the shell intact. Finely chop the scooped out zucchini flesh.

2. In a large skillet, heat the olive oil over medium heat. Add the onion and sauté for 3-4 minutes until translucent.

3. Add the garlic and chopped zucchini flesh to the skillet. Cook for 5 minutes, stirring occasionally, until the zucchini is tender.

4. Stir in the mushrooms and cook for 2-3 minutes more.

5. Add the diced tomatoes and cooked quinoa to the skillet. Season with salt and pepper.

6. Arrange the zucchini boats in a baking dish. Spoon the quinoa and vegetable mixture evenly into the zucchini shells.

7. Sprinkle the shredded vegan mozzarella cheese over the top of the stuffed zucchini boats.

8. Bake for 25-30 minutes, until the zucchini is tender and the cheese is melted.

9. Remove from oven and garnish with chopped fresh basil.

Serve the stuffed zucchini boats warm. This makes a delicious and nutritious plant-based main dish or side.

The combination of tender zucchini, savory quinoa filling, and melty vegan cheese creates a satisfying and flavorful meal.

20. Vegan Moussaka

PreparationTime: 45 minutes

Cook Time: 1 hour

Total Time: 1 hour 45 minutes

Serves: 6-8

For the Eggplant Layers:
- 2 medium eggplants, sliced into 1/2-inch rounds
- 2 tbsp olive oil
- Salt and pepper to taste

For the Lentil Meat Filling:
- 1 tbsp olive oil
- 1 onion, diced
- 3 garlic cloves, minced
- 1 cup brown or green lentils, rinsed
- 1 (14 oz) can diced tomatoes
- 1 tsp dried oregano
- 1 tsp ground cinnamon
- 1/2 tsp ground allspice
- Salt and pepper to taste

For the Béchamel Sauce:
- 3 cups unsweetened almond milk
- 1/4 cup all-purpose flour
- 2 tbsp vegan butter
- 1/4 tsp ground nutmeg
- Salt and pepper to taste

Dinner

1. Preheat oven to 400°F. Line two baking sheets with parchment paper.

2. Arrange the eggplant slices in a single layer on the prepared baking sheets. Brush both sides with olive oil and season with salt and pepper. Roast for 20-25 minutes, flipping halfway, until tender and lightly browned. Set aside.

3. In a large skillet, heat 1 tbsp olive oil over medium heat. Add the onion and sauté for 5 minutes until translucent.

4. Stir in the garlic and lentils. Cook for 2-3 minutes until fragrant.

5. Add the diced tomatoes, oregano, cinnamon, allspice, salt, and pepper. Simmer for 20-25 minutes, until the lentils are tender and the mixture has thickened.

6. In a medium saucepan, whisk together the almond milk and flour over medium heat. Bring to a simmer and cook for 5-7 minutes, stirring frequently, until thickened.

7. Remove from heat and stir in the vegan butter, nutmeg, salt, and pepper.

8. Grease a 9x13 inch baking dish. Layer half of the roasted eggplant slices in the bottom. Top with the lentil meat filling, then the remaining eggplant slices.

9. Pour the béchamel sauce evenly over the top. Bake for 30-35 minutes, until the top is golden brown. Let the moussaka stand for 10 minutes before serving.

Enjoy this hearty and flavorful vegan moussaka! The layers of roasted eggplant, savory lentil filling, and creamy béchamel sauce make for a delicious plant-based dish.

21. Roasted Cauliflower Steaks with Chimichurri Sauce

PreparationTime: 20 minutes

Cook Time: 30 minutes

Total Time: 50 minutes

Serves: 4

For the Cauliflower Steaks:
- 1 large head of cauliflower, cut into 1-inch thick slices
- 2 tbsp olive oil
- Salt and pepper to taste

For the Chimichurri Sauce:
- 1 cup packed fresh parsley
- 1/2 cup packed fresh cilantro
- 3 garlic cloves
- 2 tbsp red wine vinegar
- 1 tbsp olive oil
- 1 tsp dried oregano
- 1/4 tsp red pepper flakes
- Salt and pepper to taste

Dinner

1. Preheat oven to 400°F. Line a baking sheet with parchment paper.

2. Arrange the cauliflower slices in a single layer on the prepared baking sheet. Brush both sides with the olive oil and season with salt and pepper.

3. Roast the cauliflower for 25-30 minutes, flipping halfway, until tender and lightly browned.

4. While the cauliflower is roasting, make the chimichurri sauce. In a food processor, combine the parsley, cilantro, garlic, red wine vinegar, olive oil, oregano, and red pepper flakes. Pulse until a coarse sauce forms. Season with salt and pepper to taste.

5. Transfer the roasted cauliflower steaks to a serving platter. Drizzle the chimichurri sauce generously over the top.

6. Serve the cauliflower steaks warm, with any extra chimichurri sauce on the side.

This dish makes a delicious and impressive plant-based main or side. The tender roasted cauliflower is elevated by the bold and flavorful chimichurri sauce. Enjoy this healthy and satisfying meal!

22. Vegan Paella

PreparationTime: 30 minutes
Cook Time: 45 minutes
Total Time: 1 hour 15 minutes
Serves: 4-6

- 1 cup short-grain Spanish rice (such as Bomba or Calasparra)
- 3 cups vegetable broth
- 1 tbsp olive oil
- 1 onion, diced
- 3 garlic cloves, minced
- 1 tsp smoked paprika
- 1/2 tsp saffron threads
- 1 tsp dried thyme
- 1 cup diced tomatoes
- 1 cup frozen peas
- 1 cup sliced mushrooms
- 1 (15 oz) can artichoke hearts, drained and quartered
- 1 (15 oz) can chickpeas, drained and rinsed
- Salt and pepper to taste
- Chopped parsley for garnish

Dinner

1. In a medium saucepan, bring the vegetable broth to a simmer. Add the rice, cover, and cook for 18-20 minutes until the rice is tender. Fluff with a fork and set aside.

2. In a large paella pan or skillet, heat the olive oil over medium heat. Add the onion and sauté for 5 minutes until translucent.

3. Stir in the garlic, smoked paprika, saffron, and thyme. Cook for 1 minute until fragrant.

4. Add the diced tomatoes, peas, mushrooms, artichoke hearts, and chickpeas. Season with salt and pepper.

5. Gently fold in the cooked rice until everything is well combined.

6. Reduce heat to low, cover, and simmer for 15-20 minutes, stirring occasionally, until the rice is tender and the flavors have melded.

7. Remove from heat and let stand for 5 minutes.

8. Garnish the vegan paella with chopped parsley before serving.

Serve the paella warm, directly from the pan. This colorful and flavorful plant-based dish is a delicious and authentic-tasting version of the classic Spanish rice dish.

23. Vegan Pot Pie

PreparationTime: 45 minutes

Cook Time: 45 minutes

Total Time: 1 hour 30 minutes

Serves: 4-6

For the Filling:
- 1 tbsp olive oil
- 1 onion, diced
- 3 carrots, peeled and diced
- 3 celery stalks, diced
- 8 oz cremini mushrooms, sliced
- 3 garlic cloves, minced
- 1 tsp dried thyme
- 1 tsp dried rosemary
- 1/4 cup all-purpose flour
- 2 cups vegetable broth
- 1 (15 oz) can diced tomatoes
- 1 (15 oz) can chickpeas, drained and rinsed
- 1 cup frozen peas
- Salt and pepper to taste

For the Crust:
- 2 cups all-purpose flour
- 1 tsp salt
- 2/3 cup cold vegan butter, cubed
- 6-8 tbsp ice water

Dinner

1. Preheat oven to 400°F.

2. Make the filling: In a large skillet, heat the olive oil over medium heat. Add the onion, carrots, celery, and mushrooms. Sauté for 5-7 minutes until the vegetables are tender.

3. Stir in the garlic, thyme, and rosemary. Cook for 1 minute until fragrant.

4. Sprinkle the flour over the vegetable mixture and stir to coat. Cook for 2 minutes.

5. Gradually whisk in the vegetable broth and diced tomatoes. Bring to a simmer and cook for 5-7 minutes, until thickened.

6. Stir in the chickpeas and frozen peas. Season with salt and pepper to taste.

7. Make the crust: In a food processor, pulse the flour and salt together. Add the cold vegan butter and pulse until the mixture resembles coarse crumbs.

8. Add the ice water 1 tbsp at a time, pulsing just until the dough begins to come together. Do not overmix.

9. Turn the dough out onto a lightly floured surface and gather into a disc. Wrap in plastic and refrigerate for 30 minutes.

10. Roll out the dough to fit a 9-inch pie dish. Transfer the filling to the dish and top with the pie crust.

11. Bake for 35-40 minutes, until the crust is golden brown.

12. Let the pot pie cool for 10 minutes before serving

24. Red Lentil and Spinach Dhal

PreparationTime: 15 minutes

Cook Time: 30 minutes

Total Time: 45 minutes

Serves: 4

- 1 cup dry red lentils, rinsed
- 4 cups vegetable broth
- 1 tbsp olive oil
- 1 onion, diced
- 3 garlic cloves, minced
- 1 tbsp grated ginger
- 1 tsp ground cumin
- 1 tsp ground coriander
- 1 tsp garam masala
- 1/4 tsp cayenne pepper (or to taste)
- 1 (14 oz) can diced tomatoes
- 5 oz baby spinach
- 1 tsp lime juice
- Salt and pepper to taste
- Chopped cilantro for garnish

Dinner

1. In a large saucepan, combine the red lentils and vegetable broth. Bring to a boil, then reduce heat and simmer for 15-20 minutes, until the lentils are tender.

2. In a separate skillet, heat the olive oil over medium heat. Add the diced onion and sauté for 5 minutes until translucent.

3. Stir in the garlic, ginger, cumin, coriander, garam masala, and cayenne. Cook for 1-2 minutes until fragrant.

4. Add the diced tomatoes and their juices to the skillet. Simmer for 5 minutes.

5. Stir the cooked lentils into the tomato-spice mixture. Add the baby spinach and lime juice. Cook for 2-3 minutes, until the spinach is wilted.

6. Season the dhal with salt and pepper to taste.

7. Serve the red lentil and spinach dhal warm, garnished with chopped cilantro. Accompany with basmati rice or naan bread.

This nourishing and flavorful dhal makes a delicious plant-based main dish or side. The combination of red lentils, aromatic spices, and fresh spinach creates a comforting and satisfying meal.

25. Sweet and Sour Tofu

PreparationTime: 20 minutes

Cook Time: 20 minutes

Total Time: 40 minutes

Serves: 4

- 1 block (14 oz) extra-firm tofu, pressed and cubed
- 2 tbsp cornstarch
- 2 tbsp vegetable oil, divided
- 1 red bell pepper, diced
- 1 cup pineapple chunks
- 3 green onions, sliced
- 2 garlic cloves, minced

For the Sauce:
- 1/4 cup rice vinegar
- 2 tbsp soy sauce
- 2 tbsp ketchup
- 2 tbsp brown sugar
- 1 tbsp tomato paste
- 1 tsp sesame oil
- 1/4 tsp red pepper flakes (optional)

Dinner

1. In a shallow bowl, toss the cubed tofu with the cornstarch until evenly coated.

2. In a large skillet or wok, heat 1 tbsp of the vegetable oil over medium-high heat. Add the coated tofu cubes and cook for 5-7 minutes, turning occasionally, until golden brown on all sides. Transfer the tofu to a plate.

3. In the same skillet, heat the remaining 1 tbsp of oil. Add the diced bell pepper, pineapple chunks, green onions, and garlic. Stir-fry for 3-4 minutes until the vegetables are tender-crisp.

4. In a small bowl, whisk together all the sauce ingredients.

5. Add the cooked tofu back to the skillet with the vegetables. Pour the sauce over the top and toss everything together.

6. Bring the mixture to a simmer and cook for 5-7 minutes, stirring occasionally, until the sauce has thickened.

7. Serve the sweet and sour tofu immediately, over steamed rice if desired. Garnish with additional green onions.

This sweet, sour, and savory vegan tofu dish is a delicious plant-based take on the classic Chinese takeout favorite. The crispy tofu and fresh veggies in the tangy sauce make for a flavorful and satisfying meal.

1. Roasted Chickpeas

PreparationTime: 10 minutes
Cook Time: 25 minutes
Total Time: 35 minutes
Serves: 4

- 1 (15 oz) can chickpeas, drained and rinsed
- 1 tbsp olive oil
- 1 tsp ground cumin
- 1 tsp paprika
- 1/2 tsp garlic powder
- 1/4 tsp cayenne pepper (optional)
- Salt and pepper to taste

Snacks

1. Preheat oven to 400°F. Line a baking sheet with parchment paper.

2. Pat the drained and rinsed chickpeas dry with a paper towel or clean kitchen towel.

3. In a medium bowl, toss the chickpeas with the olive oil, cumin, paprika, garlic powder, and cayenne (if using). Season with salt and pepper.

4. Spread the seasoned chickpeas in a single layer on the prepared baking sheet.

5. Roast for 20-25 minutes, shaking the pan halfway, until the chickpeas are crispy and golden brown.

6. Remove the roasted chickpeas from the oven and let cool for 5 minutes before serving.

Enjoy the roasted chickpeas as a snack, salad topping, or addition to other dishes. The combination of spices gives them a delicious savory flavor.

These crispy roasted chickpeas are a simple and healthy plant-based option that can be customized with your favorite seasonings. They make a great high-protein, fiber-rich snack or side.

2. Veggie Sticks with Hummus

PreparationTime: 10 minutes
Cook Time: 0 minutes
Total Time: 10 minutes
Serves: 4-6 people

- Assorted fresh vegetables (such as carrot sticks, celery sticks, cucumber slices, bell pepper strips)
- 1 batch of homemade or store-bought hummus (about 1 cup)

1. Wash and prepare the vegetables. Cut them into long, thin sticks or slices.

2. Arrange the veggie sticks on a serving platter or plate.

3. Scoop the hummus into a small bowl and place it in the center of the plate with the veggie sticks.

4. Serve the veggie sticks with the hummus for dipping.

Tips:
- Try to include a variety of colorful vegetables for visual appeal.
- You can make your own hummus or use a store-bought brand.
- Serve the veggie sticks chilled or at room temperature.
- This makes a great healthy snack or appetizer.
- Feel free to experiment with different vegetable combinations.

Enjoy your fresh and nutritious Veggie Sticks with Hummus!

Snacks

3. Apple Slices with Almond Butter

PreparationTime: 5 minutes

Cook Time: 0 minutes

Total Time: 5 minutes

Serves: 1-2 people

- 1-2 apples, cored and sliced
- 2-3 tablespoons almond butter

1. Wash and core the apples. Slice them into thin wedges or slices.

2. Arrange the apple slices on a plate or serving board.

3. Scoop the almond butter into a small bowl or ramekin and place it next to the apple slices.

4. Serve the apple slices with the almond butter for dipping or spreading.

Tips:
- Choose crisp, fresh apples like Gala, Fuji, or Honeycrisp.
- You can use any nut butter you prefer, such as peanut butter or cashew butter.
- For added flavor, sprinkle a pinch of cinnamon over the apple slices.
- This makes a great healthy snack or light dessert.
- Feel free to adjust the amounts of apples and almond butter to your liking.

Enjoy your simple and nutritious Apple Slices with Almond Butter!

Snacks

4. Trail Mix with Nuts and Dried Fruit

PreparationTime: 10 minutes

Total Time: 10 minutes

Serves: 4

- 1/2 cup raw almonds
- 1/2 cup raw cashews
- 1/2 cup raw walnuts
- 1/2 cup raw pumpkin seeds
- 1/2 cup dried cranberries
- 1/2 cup dried apricots, chopped
- 1/4 cup unsweetened shredded coconut

Snacks

1. In a large bowl, combine all the ingredients - the almonds, cashews, walnuts, pumpkin seeds, dried cranberries, dried apricots, and shredded coconut.

2. Stir the ingredients together until well mixed.

3. Transfer the trail mix to an airtight container or resealable bag.

4. Store the trail mix at room temperature for up to 2 weeks.

This homemade trail mix is a nutritious and delicious snack option. The combination of crunchy nuts, chewy dried fruit, and toasted coconut provides a satisfying blend of flavors and textures.

The nuts offer healthy fats, protein, and fiber, while the dried fruit adds natural sweetness. This trail mix makes a great on-the-go snack or can be enjoyed as part of a balanced meal.

Feel free to adjust the ratios or swap in your favorite nuts and dried fruits to customize the trail mix to your taste.

5. Edamame with Sea Salt

PreparationTime: 5 minutes

Cook Time: 5 minutes

Total Time: 10 minutes

Serves: 2-3 people

- 1 pound (454g) frozen edamame in the pod
- 1 teaspoon sea salt

1. Bring a large pot of water to a boil.

2. Add the frozen edamame pods to the boiling water and cook for 5 minutes.

3. Drain the edamame and transfer them to a serving bowl.

4. Sprinkle the sea salt over the hot edamame and toss to coat evenly.

5. Serve the edamame warm, with the pods still intact.

Tips:
- You can use regular table salt if you don't have sea salt.
- For extra flavor, try adding a squeeze of lemon juice or a sprinkle of garlic powder.
- Edamame can be served as a snack, appetizer, or side dish.
- Leftovers can be stored in the refrigerator for up to 3 days.
- Reheat the edamame briefly in the microwave or in a skillet before serving.

Enjoy your simple and tasty Edamame with Sea Salt!

Snacks

6. Energy Balls with Dates and Nuts

PreparationTime: 15 minutes

Chilling Time: 30 minutes

Total Time: 45 minutes

Serves: 12–15 balls

- 1 cup (150g) pitted dates
- 1 cup (150g) mixed nuts (such as almonds, walnuts, pecans)
- 1/4 cup (35g) unsweetened shredded coconut
- 2 tablespoons nut butter (such as almond or peanut butter)
- 1 tablespoon honey or maple syrup (optional)
- 1/4 teaspoon sea salt

1. In a food processor, pulse the pitted dates until they form a sticky, paste-like consistency.

2. Add the mixed nuts to the food processor and pulse until the nuts are finely chopped and well combined with the dates.

3. Transfer the date-nut mixture to a medium bowl and stir in the shredded coconut, nut butter, honey or maple syrup (if using), and sea salt. Mix until all the ingredients are well incorporated.

4. Using your hands, roll the mixture into small, bite-sized balls, about 1-inch in diameter.

5. Place the energy balls on a parchment-lined baking sheet or plate.

6. Refrigerate the energy balls for at least 30 minutes to allow them to firm up.

7. Serve chilled or at room temperature.

Tips:
- Store the energy balls in an airtight container in the refrigerator for up to 1 week.
- You can customize the recipe by using different types of nuts, dried fruits, or add-ins like chia seeds or cocoa powder.
- These energy balls make a great healthy snack or pre-workout fuel.

Enjoy your homemade Energy Balls with Dates and Nuts!

Snacks

7. Baked Kale Chips

PreparationTime: 10 minutes

Cook Time: 12-15 minutes

Total Time: 22-25 minutes

Serves: 2-3 people

- 1 bunch of kale, washed and dried thoroughly
- 1-2 tablespoons olive oil
- 1/2 teaspoon sea salt (or to taste)

1. Preheat your oven to 350°F (175°C).

2. Wash the kale and pat it dry thoroughly with paper towels or a clean kitchen towel. Make sure the kale is completely dry, as any moisture will prevent the chips from crisping up.

3. Remove the tough stems from the kale leaves and tear or cut the leaves into bite-sized pieces.

4. Place the kale leaves in a large bowl and drizzle with the olive oil. Use your hands to massage the oil into the kale, ensuring all the leaves are evenly coated.

5. Arrange the kale leaves in a single layer on one or more baking sheets, making sure they are not overlapping.

6. Sprinkle the sea salt evenly over the kale leaves.

7. Bake for 12-15 minutes, or until the kale chips are crispy and lightly browned. Keep a close eye on them to prevent burning.

8. Remove the baked kale chips from the oven and let them cool for a few minutes before serving.

Tips:
- Experiment with different seasonings, such as garlic powder, paprika, or chili powder.
- Store any leftover kale chips in an airtight container for up to 3 days.
- Enjoy the kale chips as a healthy snack or side dish.

Bon appétit!

Snacks

8. Vegan Cheese and Crackers

PreparationTime: 10 minutes
Chilling Time: 2 hours
Total Time: 2 hours 10 minutes
Serves: 4-6 people

For the Vegan Cheese:
- 1 cup raw cashews, soaked in water for at least 2 hours
- 1/4 cup unsweetened almond milk
- 2 tablespoons lemon juice
- 1 teaspoon apple cider vinegar
- 1/2 teaspoon sea salt
- 1/4 teaspoon garlic powder
- 1/4 teaspoon onion powder

For the Crackers:
- 1 cup whole wheat crackers or gluten-free crackers of your choice

For the Vegan Cheese:
1. Drain and rinse the soaked cashews.
2. In a high-speed blender or food processor, blend the cashews, almond milk, lemon juice, apple cider vinegar, salt, garlic powder, and onion powder until smooth and creamy.
3. Transfer the cheese mixture to a small bowl or ramekin and refrigerate for at least 2 hours to allow it to firm up.

For the Crackers:
1. Arrange the crackers on a serving plate or board.

To Serve:
1. Remove the chilled vegan cheese from the refrigerator.
2. Scoop or spread the cheese onto the crackers.
3. Serve the vegan cheese and crackers immediately.

Tips:
- You can customize the vegan cheese by adding herbs, spices, or other flavorings.
- Try different types of crackers, such as whole grain, seed-based, or gluten-free options.
- For a more spreadable consistency, add a bit more almond milk to the cheese mixture.
- Store any leftover vegan cheese in an airtight container in the refrigerator for up to 5 days.

Enjoy your delicious Vegan Cheese and Crackers!

9. Fresh Fruit Salad

PreparationTime: 20 minutes

Chilling Time: 30 minutes

Total Time: 50 minutes

Serves: 4-6 people

- 1 cup diced pineapple
- 1 cup diced mango
- 1 cup halved strawberries
- 1 cup blueberries
- 1 cup diced kiwi
- 1 cup diced honeydew or cantaloupe
- 2 tablespoons freshly squeezed orange juice
- 1 tablespoon honey (optional)
- 1/4 teaspoon ground cinnamon (optional)

Snacks

1. In a large bowl, combine the diced pineapple, mango, strawberries, blueberries, kiwi, and honeydew or cantaloupe.

2. Drizzle the orange juice over the fruit and gently toss to coat.

3. If desired, add the honey and cinnamon and stir to combine.

4. Cover the fruit salad and refrigerate for at least 30 minutes to allow the flavors to meld.

5. Serve the fresh fruit salad chilled.

Tips:
- Feel free to use any combination of your favorite fresh fruits.
- You can adjust the amount of orange juice and honey to your taste.
- For a creamy fruit salad, you can fold in a dollop of plain Greek yogurt or whipped cream.
- Garnish the salad with a sprig of mint or a sprinkle of toasted coconut flakes.
- This fruit salad is a great dessert, snack, or side dish.

Enjoy your refreshing and colorful Fresh Fruit Salad!

10. Popcorn with Nutritional Yeast

PreparationTime: 5 minutes

Cook Time: 5 minutes

Total Time: 10 minutes

Serves: 2-3 people

- 1/4 cup unpopped popcorn kernels
- 2 tablespoons olive oil or coconut oil
- 2-3 tablespoons nutritional yeast
- 1/2 teaspoon sea salt (or to taste)

1. In a large pot with a tight-fitting lid, heat the oil over medium-high heat.

2. Once the oil is hot, add the unpopped popcorn kernels in a single layer. Cover the pot with the lid.

3. Allow the popcorn to pop, shaking the pot occasionally to prevent burning. Once the popping slows to 2-3 seconds between pops, remove the pot from the heat.

4. Transfer the freshly popped popcorn to a large bowl.

5. Sprinkle the nutritional yeast and sea salt over the popcorn, and toss to coat the popcorn evenly.

6. Serve the Popcorn with Nutritional Yeast warm and enjoy!

Tips:
- Use high-quality, fresh popcorn kernels for the best results.
- Adjust the amount of nutritional yeast and salt to your taste preferences.
- For extra flavor, you can also add a pinch of garlic powder, paprika, or other spices.
- Store any leftover popcorn in an airtight container for up to 3 days.
- This makes a great healthy snack or movie-watching treat.

Enjoy your delicious and nutritious Popcorn with Nutritional Yeast!

Snacks

11. Celery Sticks with Peanut Butter

PreparationTime: 5 minutes

Cook Time: 0 minutes

Total Time: 5 minutes

Serves: 1-2 people

- 2-3 celery stalks, washed and cut into 4-inch sticks
- 2-3 tablespoons peanut butter (or any nut butter of your choice)

Snacks

1. Wash the celery stalks and pat them dry with a paper towel.

2. Cut the celery stalks into 4-inch sticks.

3. Spread or spoon the peanut butter onto the celery sticks, coating them evenly.

4. Arrange the celery sticks with peanut butter on a plate or serving board.

Tips:
- You can use any type of nut butter, such as almond butter or cashew butter, if you prefer.
- For added flavor, you can sprinkle a pinch of cinnamon or a drizzle of honey on top of the peanut butter.
- This snack is a great source of fiber, protein, and healthy fats.
- It's a simple and satisfying option for a quick snack or a healthy addition to a lunchbox.
- Adjust the amounts of celery and peanut butter to your personal preference.

Enjoy your Celery Sticks with Peanut Butter!

12. Avocado and Tomato Bruschetta

PreparationTime: 15 minutes

Cook Time: 5 minutes

Total Time: 20 minutes

Serves: 4-6 people

- 1 baguette, sliced into 1/2-inch thick rounds
- 2 ripe avocados, pitted and diced
- 1 cup diced tomatoes
- 2 tablespoons finely chopped red onion
- 2 tablespoons chopped fresh basil
- 1 tablespoon olive oil
- 1 tablespoon balsamic vinegar
- 1/2 teaspoon sea salt
- 1/4 teaspoon freshly ground black pepper

Snacks

1. Preheat your oven to 400°F (200°C).

2. Arrange the baguette slices on a baking sheet. Lightly brush or drizzle the slices with a small amount of olive oil.

3. Bake the baguette slices for 5 minutes, or until lightly toasted and crispy.

4. In a medium bowl, combine the diced avocado, tomatoes, red onion, basil, olive oil, balsamic vinegar, salt, and pepper. Gently toss to mix well.

5. Top each toasted baguette slice with a spoonful of the avocado-tomato mixture.

6. Serve the avocado and tomato bruschetta immediately.

Tips:
- Use ripe, flavorful tomatoes for the best results.
- Adjust the amount of vinegar and seasoning to your taste.
- For a creamier texture, you can mash the avocado slightly before mixing with the other ingredients.
- Garnish the bruschetta with additional fresh basil leaves, if desired.
- This makes a great appetizer or light snack.

Enjoy your fresh and delicious Avocado and Tomato Bruschetta!

13. Mixed Berry Bowl

PreparationTime: 10 minutes

Chilling Time: 30 minutes (optional)

Total Time: 40 minutes

Serves: 4 people

- 1 cup fresh strawberries, hulled and halved
- 1 cup fresh blueberries
- 1 cup fresh raspberries
- 1 cup fresh blackberries
- 2 tablespoons honey or maple syrup (optional)
- 1 tablespoon freshly squeezed lemon juice
- 1/4 teaspoon ground cinnamon (optional)

Snacks

1. In a large bowl, gently combine the strawberries, blueberries, raspberries, and blackberries.

2. If desired, drizzle the honey or maple syrup over the berries and toss to coat.

3. Sprinkle the lemon juice and ground cinnamon (if using) over the mixed berries and gently stir to incorporate.

4. Cover the bowl and refrigerate for at least 30 minutes to allow the flavors to meld (optional).

5. Serve the chilled Mixed Berry Bowl as a refreshing snack, breakfast, or dessert.

Tips:
- Feel free to use any combination of fresh berries you have available.
- Adjust the amount of honey or maple syrup to your desired sweetness level.
- For a creamier texture, you can serve the Mixed Berry Bowl with a dollop of plain Greek yogurt or whipped cream.
- Garnish with a sprig of fresh mint or a sprinkle of toasted nuts or granola.
- This dish is best enjoyed within a day of preparation for the freshest flavor.

Enjoy your vibrant and healthy Mixed Berry Bowl!

14. Vegan Spinach Artichoke Dip

PreparationTime: 15 minutes

Cook Time: 20 minutes

Total Time: 35 minutes

Serves: 6-8 people

- 1 (14 oz) can artichoke hearts, drained and chopped
- 1 (10 oz) package frozen chopped spinach, thawed and drained
- 1 cup raw cashews, soaked in water for at least 2 hours
- 1/2 cup unsweetened almond milk
- 2 tablespoons lemon juice
- 1 garlic clove, minced
- 1 teaspoon Dijon mustard
- 1/2 teaspoon sea salt
- 1/4 teaspoon ground black pepper

For Serving:
- Crackers, pita chips, or fresh vegetables (such as carrot sticks, celery sticks, or cucumber slices)

Snacks

1. Preheat your oven to 375°F (190°C).

2. Drain and rinse the soaked cashews. In a high-speed blender or food processor, blend the cashews, almond milk, lemon juice, garlic, Dijon mustard, salt, and pepper until smooth and creamy.

3. In a medium bowl, combine the chopped artichoke hearts and thawed, drained spinach. Pour the cashew-based sauce over the artichoke and spinach mixture and stir to mix well.

4. Transfer the spinach artichoke dip to a baking dish or oven-safe serving bowl.

5. Bake the dip for 20-25 minutes, or until heated through and lightly browned on top.

6. Remove the dip from the oven and let it cool for a few minutes before serving.

7. Serve the warm Vegan Spinach Artichoke Dip with your choice of crackers, pita chips, or fresh vegetables.

Tips:
- For a creamier texture, add an extra 1-2 tablespoons of almond milk to the cashew-based sauce.
- Adjust the seasoning to your taste, adding more salt, pepper, or lemon juice as desired.
- This dip can be made in advance and reheated before serving.
- Store any leftover dip in an airtight container in the refrigerator for up to 4 days.

Enjoy your delicious and creamy Vegan Spinach Artichoke Dip!

15. Spicy Roasted Almonds

PreparationTime: 5 minutes

Cook Time: 15 minutes

Total Time: 20 minutes

Serves: 4 people

- 2 cups raw almonds
- 1 tablespoon olive oil
- 1 teaspoon paprika
- 1/2 teaspoon cayenne pepper
- 1/2 teaspoon garlic powder
- 1/2 teaspoon ground cumin
- 1/2 teaspoon sea salt

1. Preheat your oven to 350°F (175°C).

2. In a medium bowl, toss the raw almonds with the olive oil until the almonds are evenly coated.

3. In a small bowl, mix together the paprika, cayenne pepper, garlic powder, cumin, and sea salt.

4. Sprinkle the spice mixture over the oiled almonds and toss to coat them evenly.

5. Spread the seasoned almonds in a single layer on a baking sheet.

6. Roast the almonds in the preheated oven for 12-15 minutes, stirring halfway, until they are fragrant and lightly browned.

7. Remove the roasted almonds from the oven and let them cool for a few minutes before serving.

Tips:
- Adjust the amount of cayenne pepper to your desired level of spiciness.
- You can use any combination of spices you enjoy, such as chili powder, smoked paprika, or ground coriander.
- For extra flavor, you can add a pinch of brown sugar or maple syrup to the spice mixture.
- Store the cooled Spicy Roasted Almonds in an airtight container at room temperature for up to 1 week.
- These almonds make a great snack, topping for salads, or addition to trail mixes.

Enjoy your delicious and flavorful Spicy Roasted Almonds!

1. Vegan Chocolate Avocado Mousse

PreparationTime: 10 minutes

Chilling Time: 2 hours

Total Time: 2 hours 10 minutes

Serves: 4 people

- 2 ripe avocados, pitted and flesh scooped out
- 1/2 cup unsweetened cocoa powder
- 1/4 cup maple syrup (or agave nectar)
- 1/4 cup unsweetened almond milk
- 1 teaspoon vanilla extract
- 1/4 teaspoon sea salt

1. In a high-speed blender or food processor, combine the avocado flesh, cocoa powder, maple syrup, almond milk, vanilla extract, and sea salt. Blend until the mixture is smooth and creamy, scraping down the sides as needed.

2. Divide the chocolate avocado mousse evenly into 4 small serving bowls or ramekins.

3. Cover the bowls with plastic wrap or transfer the mousse to an airtight container.

4. Refrigerate the vegan chocolate avocado mousse for at least 2 hours, or until it has set and thickened.

5. Serve the chilled mousse garnished with fresh berries, shredded coconut, or a sprinkle of cocoa powder, if desired.

Tips:
- Use very ripe, soft avocados for the best texture.
- Adjust the sweetness to your taste by adding more or less maple syrup.
- For a thicker consistency, use less almond milk.
- This mousse can be made a day in advance and stored in the refrigerator.
- Leftovers will keep in the fridge for up to 3 days.

Enjoy your rich and creamy Vegan Chocolate Avocado Mousse!

Desserts

2. Chia Seed Pudding with Mango

PreparationTime: 10 minutes

Chilling Time: 4 hours

Total Time: 4 hours 10 minutes

Serves: 4 people

- 1/2 cup chia seeds
- 2 cups unsweetened almond milk (or any plant-based milk)
- 2 tablespoons maple syrup (or honey)
- 1 teaspoon vanilla extract
- 1 ripe mango, peeled and diced
- Mint leaves for garnish (optional)

1. In a medium bowl, whisk together the chia seeds, almond milk, maple syrup, and vanilla extract until well combined.

2. Cover the bowl and refrigerate for at least 4 hours, or overnight, stirring occasionally, until the chia seeds have thickened the mixture into a pudding-like consistency.

3. Once the chia seed pudding has set, divide it evenly into 4 serving bowls or glasses.

4. Top each portion of chia seed pudding with a generous amount of diced mango.

5. Garnish with fresh mint leaves, if desired.

6. Serve the Chia Seed Pudding with Mango chilled.

Tips:
- For a creamier texture, use full-fat coconut milk instead of almond milk.
- Adjust the sweetness by adding more or less maple syrup or honey to your taste.
- Try using other fresh fruits, such as berries or pineapple, in place of the mango.
- This pudding can be made a day in advance and stored in the refrigerator.
- The chia seed pudding will keep for up to 4 days in the fridge.

Enjoy your delicious and nutritious Chia Seed Pudding with Mango!

Desserts

3. Baked Apples with Cinnamon

PreparationTime: 10 minutes

Cook Time: 30 minutes

Total Time: 40 minutes

Serves: 4 people

- 4 medium-sized apples (such as Gala, Honeycrisp, or Fuji)
- 1/4 cup brown sugar
- 1 teaspoon ground cinnamon
- 2 tablespoons unsalted butter, softened
- 1/4 cup chopped walnuts or pecans (optional)
- Vanilla ice cream or whipped cream (optional, for serving)

Desserts

1. Preheat your oven to 375°F (190°C).

2. Wash and core the apples, leaving a small well in the center of each one. Be careful not to cut all the way through.

3. In a small bowl, mix together the brown sugar and cinnamon.

4. Stuff the brown sugar-cinnamon mixture into the center of each apple. Top each apple with a small pat of the softened butter.

5. Place the stuffed apples in a baking dish or on a rimmed baking sheet.

6. Bake for 30-35 minutes, or until the apples are tender and the filling is bubbly.

7. Remove the baked apples from the oven and let them cool for a few minutes.

8. Serve the Baked Apples with Cinnamon warm, optionally topped with a scoop of vanilla ice cream or a dollop of whipped cream.

Tips:
- For extra flavor, you can add a sprinkle of chopped walnuts or pecans to the filling.
- Adjust the baking time if using larger or smaller apples.
- Leftovers can be stored in the refrigerator for up to 3 days and reheated before serving.

Enjoy your delicious and comforting Baked Apples with Cinnamon!

4. Vegan Banana Bread

PreparationTime: 15 minutes

Cook Time: 55-60 minutes

Total Time: 1 hour 10 minutes

Serves: 8-10 slices

- 3 ripe bananas, mashed (about 1 cup)
- 1/3 cup unsweetened applesauce
- 1/2 cup maple syrup or agave nectar
- 1/4 cup unsweetened almond milk
- 1 teaspoon vanilla extract
- 1 3/4 cups all-purpose flour (or gluten-free flour blend)
- 1 teaspoon baking soda
- 1/2 teaspoon ground cinnamon
- 1/4 teaspoon sea salt
- 1/2 cup chopped walnuts or pecans (optional)

Desserts

1. Preheat your oven to 350°F (175°C). Grease a 9x5-inch loaf pan with non-stick cooking spray or line it with parchment paper.

2. In a medium bowl, mash the ripe bananas until smooth. Add the applesauce, maple syrup, almond milk, and vanilla extract, and stir to combine.

3. In a separate bowl, whisk together the flour, baking soda, cinnamon, and salt.

4. Slowly add the dry ingredients to the wet ingredients, mixing just until combined. Do not overmix.

5. If using, fold in the chopped walnuts or pecans.

6. Pour the batter into the prepared loaf pan and smooth the top.

7. Bake for 55-60 minutes, or until a toothpick inserted into the center comes out clean.

8. Allow the vegan banana bread to cool in the pan for 10 minutes, then transfer it to a wire rack to cool completely before slicing.

Tips:
- For a moister bread, use very ripe, spotty bananas.
- Substitute the all-purpose flour with whole wheat flour or a gluten-free blend for a healthier option.
- Add chocolate chips, dried fruit, or other mix-ins to customize the bread.
- Serve the vegan banana bread sliced, with a spread of nut butter or vegan cream cheese, if desired.
- Store the cooled bread in an airtight container at room temperature for up to 4 days, or freeze for up to 3 months.

Enjoy your delicious and moist Vegan Banana Bread!

5. Coconut Yogurt with Fresh Berries

PreparationTime: 5 minutes

Chilling Time: 30 minutes (optional)

Total Time: 35 minutes

Serves: 2 people

- 1 cup unsweetened coconut yogurt
- 1 cup mixed fresh berries (such as raspberries, blueberries, and strawberries)
- 1 tablespoon honey or maple syrup (optional)
- 1 teaspoon vanilla extract (optional)

1. In a medium bowl, scoop out the coconut yogurt.

2. Gently fold in the mixed fresh berries, being careful not to crush the berries.

3. If desired, drizzle the honey or maple syrup over the coconut yogurt and berries, and add the vanilla extract. Stir to combine.

4. Cover the bowl and refrigerate for at least 30 minutes to allow the flavors to meld (optional).

5. Serve the Coconut Yogurt with Fresh Berries chilled.

Tips:
- Use a high-quality, unsweetened coconut yogurt for the best flavor.
- Adjust the amount of honey or maple syrup to your desired sweetness level.
- Feel free to use any combination of fresh berries you have available.
- For a creamier texture, you can use full-fat coconut milk or coconut cream instead of yogurt.
- This makes a great breakfast, snack, or light dessert.
- Leftovers can be stored in the refrigerator for up to 3 days.

Enjoy your refreshing and nutritious Coconut Yogurt with Fresh Berries!

Desserts

6. Dark Chocolate and Nut Bark

PreparationTime: 10 minutes
Chilling Time: 30 minutes
Total Time: 40 minutes
Serves: 8-10 people

- 12 oz (340g) dark chocolate, chopped (or use dark chocolate chips)
- 1/2 cup mixed nuts (such as almonds, cashews, and pecans), chopped
- 2 tablespoons unsweetened shredded coconut (optional)
- 1 teaspoon sea salt (optional)

1. Line a baking sheet or large plate with parchment paper.

2. In a double boiler or a heatproof bowl set over a saucepan of simmering water, melt the chopped dark chocolate, stirring occasionally, until smooth and completely melted.

3. Remove the melted chocolate from the heat and stir in the chopped mixed nuts.

4. Spread the chocolate-nut mixture evenly onto the prepared baking sheet or plate.

5. If using, sprinkle the shredded coconut and sea salt over the top of the chocolate bark.

6. Refrigerate the bark for at least 30 minutes, or until it has completely hardened.

7. Once set, break or cut the dark chocolate and nut bark into irregular pieces.

8. Serve the Dark Chocolate and Nut Bark at room temperature or chilled.

Tips:
- Use a high-quality dark chocolate with at least 70% cacao content for the best flavor.
- Feel free to use any combination of nuts, such as almonds, walnuts, pistachios, or hazelnuts.
- For added texture, you can also add a sprinkle of crushed graham crackers or crushed pretzels.
- Store the bark in an airtight container in the refrigerator for up to 2 weeks.
- This makes a great homemade gift or a delicious snack.

Enjoy your indulgent Dark Chocolate and Nut Bark!

Desserts

7. Vegan Lemon Bars

PreparationTime: 20 minutes

Cook Time: 30 minutes

Total Time: 50 minutes

Serves: 16 bars

For the Crust:
- 1 1/2 cups all-purpose flour
- 1/2 cup powdered sugar
- 1/2 cup vegan butter, chilled and cubed

For the Filling:
- 1 cup freshly squeezed lemon juice (about 4-5 lemons)
- 1 cup granulated sugar
- 1/2 cup aquafaba (liquid from a can of chickpeas)
- 1/4 cup all-purpose flour
- 1/4 teaspoon salt

Desserts

1. Preheat the oven to 350°F (175°C). Line an 8x8 inch baking pan with parchment paper, leaving some overhang on the sides for easy removal.

2. Make the crust: In a food processor, combine the flour, powdered sugar, and vegan butter. Pulse until the mixture resembles coarse crumbs. Press the mixture evenly into the prepared baking pan.

3. Bake the crust for 15 minutes, or until lightly golden. Remove from the oven and let cool.

4. Make the filling: In a medium bowl, whisk together the lemon juice, granulated sugar, aquafaba, flour, and salt until well combined.

5. Pour the filling over the cooled crust and spread it evenly.

6. Bake for 30 minutes, or until the filling is set. Allow the bars to cool completely in the pan, then refrigerate for at least 2 hours or overnight.

7. Once chilled, lift the bars out of the pan using the parchment paper overhang. Cut into 16 squares and dust with powdered sugar before serving.

Enjoy your delicious vegan lemon bars!

8. Apple Crisp with Oat Topping

PreparationTime: 20 minutes

Cook Time: 40 minutes

Total Time: 1 hour

Serves: 6-8

For the Filling:
- 6 cups peeled, cored, and sliced apples (about 6-8 medium apples)
- 1/2 cup granulated sugar
- 2 tablespoons all-purpose flour
- 1 teaspoon ground cinnamon
- 1/4 teaspoon ground nutmeg

For the Topping:
- 1 cup old-fashioned rolled oats
- 1/2 cup all-purpose flour
- 1/2 cup packed brown sugar
- 1/2 cup vegan butter, chilled and cubed
- 1/2 teaspoon ground cinnamon
- 1/4 teaspoon salt

Desserts

1. Preheat the oven to 350°F (175°C). Grease an 8x8 inch baking dish.

2. Make the filling: In a large bowl, toss the sliced apples with the granulated sugar, 2 tablespoons flour, 1 teaspoon cinnamon, and nutmeg. Transfer the apple mixture to the prepared baking dish.

3. Make the topping: In a medium bowl, combine the rolled oats, 1/2 cup flour, brown sugar, vegan butter, 1/2 teaspoon cinnamon, and salt. Use your fingers or a fork to mix until the mixture resembles coarse crumbs.

4. Sprinkle the oat topping evenly over the apple filling.

5. Bake for 40-45 minutes, or until the apples are tender and the topping is golden brown.

6. Allow the apple crisp to cool for at least 15 minutes before serving. Serve warm, with a scoop of vegan vanilla ice cream or whipped cream, if desired.

Enjoy your delicious Apple Crisp with Oat Topping!

9. Vegan Chocolate Chip Cookies

PreparationTime: 15 minutes

Bake Time: 12-15 minutes

Total Time: 27-30 minutes

Yields: 18-20 cookies

- 1 1/4 cups all-purpose flour
- 1/2 teaspoon baking soda
- 1/4 teaspoon salt
- 1/2 cup vegan butter, softened
- 3/4 cup brown sugar
- 1/4 cup unsweetened applesauce
- 1 teaspoon vanilla extract
- 1 cup vegan chocolate chips

1. Preheat your oven to 350°F (175°C). Line a baking sheet with parchment paper.

2. In a medium bowl, whisk together the all-purpose flour, baking soda, and salt. Set aside.

3. In a large bowl, cream the softened vegan butter and brown sugar together until light and fluffy, about 2-3 minutes.

4. Add the unsweetened applesauce and vanilla extract to the butter mixture and mix until well combined.

5. Gradually add the dry ingredients to the wet ingredients, mixing just until a dough forms. Fold in the vegan chocolate chips.

6. Scoop the dough by the tablespoonful and place them about 2 inches apart on the prepared baking sheet.

7. Bake for 12-15 minutes, or until the edges are lightly golden brown.

8. Remove the cookies from the oven and let them cool on the baking sheet for 5 minutes before transferring them to a wire rack to cool completely.

Tips:
- Use room temperature vegan butter for best results.
- Substitute the all-purpose flour with a gluten-free flour blend for a gluten-free version.
- Try using a mix of dark chocolate and milk chocolate chips for variety.
- For chewier cookies, bake for the shorter end of the time range.
- Store the cooled cookies in an airtight container at room temperature for up to 5 days.

Enjoy your delicious and chewy Vegan Chocolate Chip Cookies!

Desserts

10. Raspberry Chia Jam Bars

PreparationTime: 20 minutes

Cook Time: 30 minutes

Total Time: 50 minutes

Serves: 16 bars

For the Crust:
- 1 1/2 cups all-purpose flour
- 1/2 cup rolled oats
- 1/2 cup vegan butter, chilled and cubed
- 1/4 cup maple syrup
- 1/4 teaspoon salt

For the Raspberry Chia Jam:
- 2 cups fresh or frozen raspberries
- 1/4 cup maple syrup
- 2 tablespoons chia seeds

1. Preheat the oven to 350°F (175°C). Line an 8x8 inch baking pan with parchment paper, leaving some overhang on the sides for easy removal.

2. Make the crust: In a food processor, combine the flour, rolled oats, vegan butter, maple syrup, and salt. Pulse until the mixture resembles coarse crumbs. Press the mixture evenly into the prepared baking pan.

3. Bake the crust for 15 minutes, or until lightly golden. Remove from the oven and let cool.

4. Make the raspberry chia jam: In a medium saucepan, combine the raspberries and maple syrup. Cook over medium heat, stirring occasionally, until the raspberries have broken down and the mixture is thickened, about 10 minutes.

5. Remove the raspberry mixture from the heat and stir in the chia seeds. Let the jam cool for 5 minutes, then spread it evenly over the cooled crust.

6. Bake the bars for an additional 15 minutes, or until the jam is set.

7. Allow the bars to cool completely in the pan, then refrigerate for at least 2 hours or overnight.

8. Once chilled, lift the bars out of the pan using the parchment paper overhang. Cut into 16 squares and serve.

Enjoy your delicious Raspberry Chia Jam Bars!

Desserts

1. Stuffed Bell Peppers with Lentils and Rice

PreparationTime: 20 minutes

Cook Time: 45 minutes

Total Time: 1 hour 5 minutes

Serves: 4-6 people

- 6 medium bell peppers (any color)
- 1 cup cooked brown rice
- 1 cup cooked lentils
- 1 small onion, finely chopped
- 2 cloves garlic, minced
- 1 (14.5 oz) can diced tomatoes
- 1 teaspoon dried oregano
- 1 teaspoon ground cumin
- 1/2 teaspoon smoked paprika
- 1/4 teaspoon red pepper flakes (optional)
- Salt and black pepper to taste
- 1/2 cup shredded vegan cheese (optional)

Vegetarian/Vegan

1. Preheat your oven to 375°F (190°C).

2. Cut the tops off the bell peppers and remove the seeds and membranes. Place the hollowed-out peppers in a baking dish.

3. In a large bowl, combine the cooked rice, lentils, onion, garlic, diced tomatoes, oregano, cumin, smoked paprika, and red pepper flakes (if using). Season with salt and black pepper to taste.

4. Spoon the lentil and rice mixture evenly into the hollowed-out bell peppers.

5. If using, sprinkle the shredded vegan cheese over the top of the stuffed peppers.

6. Cover the baking dish with foil and bake for 30 minutes.

7. Remove the foil and continue baking for an additional 15 minutes, or until the peppers are tender and the filling is heated through.

8. Serve the Stuffed Bell Peppers with Lentils and Rice warm.

Tips:
- You can use any color of bell peppers for this recipe.
- Adjust the spices and seasonings to your taste preferences.
- For a heartier meal, serve the stuffed peppers with a side salad or crusty bread.
- Leftovers can be stored in the refrigerator for up to 3 days.

Enjoy your delicious and nutritious Stuffed Bell Peppers with Lentils and Rice!

2. Vegan Lentil Soup

PreparationTime: 15 minutes

Cook Time: 45 minutes

Total Time: 1 hour

Serves: 6-8 people

- 1 tablespoon olive oil
- 1 onion, diced
- 3 cloves garlic, minced
- 2 carrots, peeled and diced
- 2 celery stalks, diced
- 1 cup dried brown or green lentils, rinsed
- 6 cups vegetable broth
- 1 (14.5 oz) can diced tomatoes
- 2 teaspoons dried thyme
- 1 teaspoon dried oregano
- 1/2 teaspoon smoked paprika
- Salt and black pepper to taste
- Chopped fresh parsley for garnish (optional)

Vegetarian/Vegan

1. In a large pot or Dutch oven, heat the olive oil over medium heat.

2. Add the diced onion and sauté for 3-4 minutes until translucent.

3. Stir in the minced garlic, diced carrots, and diced celery. Cook for an additional 2-3 minutes.

4. Add the rinsed lentils, vegetable broth, diced tomatoes, dried thyme, dried oregano, and smoked paprika. Season with salt and black pepper to taste.

5. Bring the soup to a boil, then reduce the heat to low, cover, and simmer for 35-40 minutes, or until the lentils are tender.

6. Taste and adjust the seasoning as needed.

7. Serve the vegan lentil soup hot, garnished with chopped fresh parsley if desired.

Tips:
- Use brown or green lentils for a heartier texture. Red lentils will break down more and create a creamier soup.
- For a thicker soup, you can mash some of the lentils against the side of the pot with the back of a spoon.
- Add diced potatoes, spinach, or kale for extra nutrition and flavor.
- Serve the lentil soup with crusty bread or a side salad for a complete meal.
- Leftovers can be stored in the refrigerator for up to 5 days or frozen for up to 3 months.

Enjoy your comforting and nourishing Vegan Lentil Soup!

3. Roasted Vegetable Medley

PreparationTime: 20 minutes

Cook Time: 40 minutes

Total Time: 1 hour

Serves: 4-6 people

- 1 medium sweet potato, peeled and cubed
- 1 medium zucchini, sliced
- 1 red bell pepper, chopped
- 1 cup Brussels sprouts, halved
- 1 red onion, sliced
- 3 cloves garlic, minced
- 2 tablespoons olive oil
- 1 teaspoon dried thyme
- 1 teaspoon dried rosemary
- 1/2 teaspoon smoked paprika
- Salt and black pepper to taste

1. Preheat your oven to 400°F (200°C). Line a large baking sheet with parchment paper.

2. In a large bowl, combine the cubed sweet potato, sliced zucchini, chopped bell pepper, halved Brussels sprouts, and sliced red onion.

3. Add the minced garlic, olive oil, dried thyme, dried rosemary, and smoked paprika. Season with salt and black pepper to taste. Toss everything together until the vegetables are evenly coated.

4. Spread the seasoned vegetables in a single layer on the prepared baking sheet.

5. Roast the vegetables in the preheated oven for 35-40 minutes, or until they are tender and lightly browned, stirring halfway through the cooking time.

6. Remove the roasted vegetable medley from the oven and serve hot.

Tips:
- Feel free to use any combination of your favorite vegetables, such as carrots, cauliflower, or eggplant.
- Adjust the seasoning to your taste preferences, adding more or less of the herbs and spices.
- For extra crispiness, roast the vegetables at a higher temperature (425°F/220°C) for a shorter time.
- Serve the Roasted Vegetable Medley as a side dish or as a main course over quinoa or rice.
- Leftovers can be stored in the refrigerator for up to 4 days and reheated before serving.

Enjoy your delicious and nutritious Roasted Vegetable Medley!

Vegetarian/Vegan

4. Vegan Tacos with Black Beans

PreparationTime: 20 minutes

Cook Time: 15 minutes

Total Time: 35 minutes

Serves: 4 people (2 tacos each)

- 1 (15 oz) can black beans, drained and rinsed
- 1 tablespoon olive oil
- 1 onion, diced
- 3 cloves garlic, minced
- 1 teaspoon ground cumin
- 1 teaspoon chili powder
- 1/2 teaspoon smoked paprika
- Salt and black pepper to taste
- 8-10 small corn or flour tortillas, warmed
- Toppings: shredded lettuce, diced tomatoes, sliced avocado, chopped cilantro, vegan sour cream or cashew cream

Vegetarian/Vegan

1. In a medium saucepan, heat the olive oil over medium heat. Add the diced onion and sauté for 3-4 minutes until translucent.

2. Stir in the minced garlic and cook for an additional minute until fragrant.

3. Add the drained and rinsed black beans, ground cumin, chili powder, and smoked paprika. Season with salt and black pepper to taste.

4. Mash about half of the black beans with a potato masher or the back of a fork, leaving the other half whole.

5. Cook the black bean mixture for 5-7 minutes, stirring occasionally, until heated through and the flavors have melded.

6. Warm the corn or flour tortillas according to the package Directions.

7. To assemble the tacos, place a spoonful of the black bean mixture into each warm tortilla. Top with your desired toppings, such as shredded lettuce, diced tomatoes, sliced avocado, chopped cilantro, and vegan sour cream or cashew cream.

8. Serve the Vegan Tacos with Black Beans immediately.

Tips:
- For a creamier texture, you can blend a portion of the black beans before adding them to the pan.
- Customize the toppings to your liking, such as adding shredded vegan cheese, pickled onions, or diced jalapeños.
- Serve the tacos with a side of rice, roasted vegetables, or a fresh salad for a more complete meal.
- Leftovers can be stored in the refrigerator for up to 3 days.

5. Stuffed Eggplant with Quinoa

PreparationTime: 15 minutes

Cook Time: 30 minutes

Total Time: 45 minutes

Serves: 4

- 2 medium eggplants, halved lengthwise
- 1 cup cooked quinoa
- 1/2 cup diced tomatoes
- 1/4 cup crumbled feta cheese
- 2 tbsp chopped fresh parsley
- 1 tbsp olive oil
- 1 garlic clove, minced
- Salt and pepper to taste

Vegetarian/Vegan

1. Preheat oven to 400°F. Scoop out the flesh from the eggplant halves, leaving about 1/4 inch of flesh attached to the skin. Chop the scooped out eggplant flesh.

2. In a bowl, combine the chopped eggplant flesh, quinoa, tomatoes, feta, parsley, olive oil, and garlic. Season with salt and pepper.

3. Stuff the eggplant halves evenly with the quinoa mixture.

4. Place the stuffed eggplant halves on a baking sheet. Bake for 25-30 minutes, until the eggplant is tender.

5. Serve the stuffed eggplant warm.

Enjoy this delicious and healthy vegetarian main dish!

6. Vegan Mushroom Risotto

PreparationTime: 15 minutes

Cook Time: 30 minutes

Total Time: 45 minutes

Serves: 4 people

- 1 cup arborio rice
- 4 cups vegetable broth, heated and kept warm
- 1 tablespoon olive oil
- 1 onion, finely chopped
- 3 cloves garlic, minced
- 8 oz (225g) cremini or button mushrooms, sliced
- 1/2 cup dry white wine (or additional vegetable broth)
- 1/4 cup unsweetened almond milk
- 2 tablespoons nutritional yeast
- 1 teaspoon dried thyme
- Salt and black pepper to taste
- Chopped fresh parsley for garnish (optional)

1. In a medium saucepan, bring the vegetable broth to a simmer and keep it warm over low heat.

2. In a large skillet or Dutch oven, heat the olive oil over medium heat. Add the chopped onion and sauté for 3-4 minutes until translucent.

3. Add the minced garlic and sliced mushrooms to the skillet. Cook for 5-7 minutes, stirring occasionally, until the mushrooms are tender and lightly browned.

4. Add the arborio rice to the skillet and stir to coat the grains with the oil. Cook for 2-3 minutes, stirring constantly, to toast the rice.

5. Pour in the white wine (or additional vegetable broth) and stir, scraping up any browned bits from the bottom of the skillet. Cook until the liquid is mostly absorbed, about 2-3 minutes.

6. Ladle in about 1/2 cup of the warm vegetable broth and stir constantly until the liquid is absorbed. Continue this process, adding 1/2 cup of broth at a time and stirring constantly, until the rice is tender and creamy, about 25-30 minutes total.

7. Stir in the unsweetened almond milk, nutritional yeast, and dried thyme. Season with salt and black pepper to taste.

8. Serve the vegan mushroom risotto warm, garnished with chopped fresh parsley if desired.

Tips:
- Use a variety of mushrooms for more complex flavor.
- Adjust the amount of broth and cooking time as needed to achieve the desired creamy texture.
- For a richer risotto, you can stir in a tablespoon of vegan butter or olive oil at the end.
- Leftovers can be stored in the refrigerator for up to 4 days.

7. Chickpea and Spinach Stew

PreparationTime: 15 minutes

Cook Time: 30 minutes

Total Time: 45 minutes

Serves: 4

- 1 tbsp olive oil
- 1 onion, diced
- 3 garlic cloves, minced
- 1 tsp ground cumin
- 1 tsp paprika
- 1/4 tsp cayenne pepper (optional)
- 1 (15oz) can chickpeas, drained and rinsed
- 1 (14oz) can diced tomatoes
- 4 cups vegetable broth
- 5 oz baby spinach
- Salt and pepper to taste
- Chopped cilantro for garnish (optional)

Vegetarian/Vegan

1. In a large pot or Dutch oven, heat the olive oil over medium heat. Add the onion and sauté for 5 minutes until translucent.

2. Add the garlic, cumin, paprika, and cayenne (if using). Cook for 1 minute until fragrant.

3. Stir in the chickpeas, diced tomatoes, and vegetable broth. Bring to a simmer and let cook for 20 minutes.

4. Add the baby spinach and cook for 5 more minutes until the spinach is wilted.

5. Season with salt and pepper to taste.

6. Serve the chickpea and spinach stew hot, garnished with chopped cilantro if desired.

This hearty, flavorful stew is packed with protein from the chickpeas and nutrients from the spinach. It makes a delicious and comforting vegetarian meal.

8. Vegan Vegetable Stir-Fry

PreparationTime: 20 minutes
Cook Time: 15 minutes
Total Time: 35 minutes
Serves: 4

- 2 tbsp sesame oil
- 1 red bell pepper, sliced
- 1 cup broccoli florets
- 1 cup sliced mushrooms
- 1 cup snow peas
- 1 cup shredded cabbage
- 3 garlic cloves, minced
- 1 tbsp grated fresh ginger
- 2 tbsp low-sodium soy sauce or tamari
- 1 tbsp rice vinegar
- 1 tsp sesame seeds (optional)
- Salt and pepper to taste

1. Heat the sesame oil in a large skillet or wok over high heat.

2. Add the bell pepper, broccoli, mushrooms, snow peas, and cabbage. Stir-fry for 5-7 minutes, until the vegetables are tender-crisp.

3. Add the garlic and ginger and cook for 1 minute, stirring constantly, until fragrant.

4. Pour in the soy sauce and rice vinegar. Toss everything together and cook for 2-3 more minutes.

5. Remove from heat and sprinkle with sesame seeds, if using. Season with salt and pepper to taste.

6. Serve the vegan vegetable stir-fry immediately, over rice or noodles if desired.

This colorful and flavorful stir-fry is packed with fresh vegetables and a delicious soy-ginger sauce. It's a quick and easy vegan meal that's perfect for busy weeknights.

Vegetarian/Vegan

9. Roasted Sweet Potato and Black Bean Burritos

PreparationTime: 20 minutes

Cook Time: 40 minutes

Total Time: 1 hour

Serves: 4 (makes 8 burritos)

- 2 medium sweet potatoes, peeled and cubed
- 1 tbsp olive oil
- 1 tsp chili powder
- 1/2 tsp cumin
- Salt and pepper to taste
- 1 (15oz) can black beans, drained and rinsed
- 1/2 cup salsa
- 1/4 cup chopped cilantro
- 8 large whole wheat tortillas
- 1 cup shredded cheddar or monterey jack cheese

1. Preheat oven to 400°F. Toss the cubed sweet potatoes with olive oil, chili powder, cumin, salt and pepper. Spread on a baking sheet and roast for 30-35 minutes, until tender.

2. In a bowl, mash the black beans slightly. Stir in the salsa and chopped cilantro.

3. To assemble the burritos, place a tortilla on a flat surface. Spoon 1/4 cup of the roasted sweet potatoes down the center. Top with 2-3 tbsp of the black bean mixture and 2 tbsp of shredded cheese.

4. Fold the bottom of the tortilla up over the filling, then fold in the sides and continue rolling up tightly into a burrito shape.

5. Place the burritos seam-side down on a baking sheet. Bake for 10 minutes to seal the burritos.

6. Serve the roasted sweet potato and black bean burritos warm.

These hearty, veggie-packed burritos make a delicious and satisfying meatless meal. Customize with your favorite toppings!

Vegetarian/Vegan

10. Grilled Vegetable Kabobs

PreparationTime: 20 minutes

Cook Time: 15 minutes

Total Time: 35 minutes

Serves: 4

- 1 red bell pepper, cut into 1-inch pieces
- 1 yellow bell pepper, cut into 1-inch pieces
- 1 zucchini, cut into 1-inch rounds
- 1 yellow squash, cut into 1-inch rounds
- 1 red onion, cut into 1-inch pieces
- 8 oz cremini mushrooms, halved
- 2 tbsp olive oil
- 2 tsp balsamic vinegar
- 1 tsp dried oregano
- 1 tsp dried basil
- Salt and pepper to taste

Vegetarian/Vegan

1. Preheat grill to medium-high heat.

2. In a large bowl, combine the cut vegetables - bell peppers, zucchini, yellow squash, red onion, and mushrooms.

3. Drizzle the vegetables with olive oil and balsamic vinegar. Sprinkle with dried oregano, dried basil, salt, and pepper. Toss to coat evenly.

4. Thread the seasoned vegetables onto skewers, leaving a little space between each piece.

5. Grill the vegetable kabobs for 12-15 minutes, turning occasionally, until the vegetables are tender and lightly charred.

6. Serve the grilled vegetable kabobs immediately, while hot.

These colorful and flavorful grilled veggie kabobs make a great side dish or light main course. Feel free to use your favorite seasonal vegetables.

1. Green Tea with Lemon

PreparationTime: 5 minutes

Cook Time: 5 minutes

Total Time: 10 minutes

Serves: 1

- 1 green tea bag
- 1 cup hot water (around 180°F)
- 1 tbsp freshly squeezed lemon juice
- 1 tsp honey (optional)

1. Bring 1 cup of water to a near boil, around 180°F. This temperature is ideal for brewing green tea without burning the delicate leaves.

2. Place the green tea bag in a mug or teapot. Pour the hot water over the tea bag.

3. Let the tea steep for 2-3 minutes. This allows the full flavor of the green tea to infuse the water.

4. Remove the tea bag and stir in the freshly squeezed lemon juice.

5. If desired, add 1 tsp of honey to sweeten the tea.

6. Enjoy the green tea with lemon while hot.

The bright, citrusy flavor of the lemon pairs beautifully with the earthy, grassy notes of the green tea. This refreshing beverage can be enjoyed hot or chilled over ice.

Beverages

2. Turmeric Golden Milk

PreparationTime: 5 minutes

Cook Time: 10 minutes

Total Time: 15 minutes

Serves: 1

- 1 cup unsweetened almond milk (or milk of your choice)
- 1 tsp ground turmeric
- 1/2 tsp ground ginger
- 1/4 tsp ground cinnamon
- 1 tbsp honey (or maple syrup)
- Pinch of black pepper

1. In a small saucepan, whisk together the almond milk, turmeric, ginger, cinnamon, and black pepper.

2. Heat the mixture over medium heat, whisking frequently, until it starts to steam and bubble slightly, about 5-7 minutes. Do not let it boil.

3. Remove the saucepan from the heat and stir in the honey (or maple syrup) until dissolved.

4. Pour the golden milk into a mug and enjoy immediately while hot.

Optionally, you can use a milk frother or blender to create a foamy texture before serving.

The combination of turmeric, ginger, and cinnamon gives this golden milk a warm, earthy, and slightly sweet flavor. The black pepper helps enhance the absorption of turmeric's active compound, curcumin. This comforting beverage is perfect for sipping any time of day.

Beverages

3. Fresh Mint Herbal Tea

PreparationTime: 5 minutes

Steep Time: 5-7 minutes

Total Time: 10-12 minutes

Serves: 1

- 6-8 fresh mint leaves
- 1 cup boiling water
- 1 tsp honey (optional)

1. Rinse the fresh mint leaves under cold water and pat dry.

2. Place the mint leaves in a teapot or heatproof mug.

3. Bring 1 cup of water to a boil and pour it over the mint leaves.

4. Allow the tea to steep for 5-7 minutes, allowing the mint flavor to infuse the water.

5. Strain the tea leaves out, if using a teapot.

6. Stir in 1 tsp of honey, if desired, to sweeten the tea.

7. Serve the fresh mint tea hot.

You can also chill the tea and serve it over ice for a refreshing iced mint tea.

The bright, aromatic flavor of the fresh mint leaves makes this a soothing and invigorating herbal tea. It's naturally caffeine-free and can be enjoyed any time of day.

Beverages

4. Berry Smoothie with Almond Milk

PreparationTime: 5 minutes

Blend Time: 1 minute

Total Time: 6 minutes

Serves: 1

- 1 cup unsweetened almond milk
- 1 cup frozen mixed berries (such as strawberries, blueberries, raspberries)
- 1 banana, frozen
- 1 tbsp honey (optional)
- 1 tsp chia seeds (optional)

1. Add the almond milk, frozen mixed berries, and frozen banana to a high-powered blender.

2. Blend on high speed for 1-2 minutes until the smoothie is smooth and creamy.

3. If desired, add 1 tbsp of honey to sweeten the smoothie. Blend again briefly to incorporate.

4. Sprinkle 1 tsp of chia seeds on top of the smoothie, if using.

5. Pour the berry smoothie into a glass and enjoy immediately.

The combination of sweet berries, creamy banana, and nutty almond milk makes this a delicious and nutritious smoothie. The chia seeds add a boost of fiber, protein, and healthy omega-3s.

This smoothie is perfect for a quick breakfast, snack, or anytime you need a refreshing and energizing drink. Feel free to adjust the ingredients to your taste preferences.

Beverages

5. Detox Green Juice

PreparationTime: 10 minutes
Juicing Time: 5 minutes
Total Time: 15 minutes
Serves: 1 (makes about 12 oz of juice)

- 2 cups kale, stems removed
- 1 cup spinach
- 1 green apple, cored
- 1 cucumber
- 1 inch piece fresh ginger, peeled
- 1 lemon, peeled

1. Wash all the produce thoroughly.

2. Run the kale, spinach, green apple, cucumber, ginger, and lemon through a juicer according to the manufacturer's Directions.

3. Stir or shake the juice to combine all the ingredients.

4. Pour the detox green juice into a glass and enjoy immediately.

This nutrient-dense green juice is packed with vitamins, minerals, and antioxidants from the leafy greens, apple, cucumber, ginger, and lemon. The ginger and lemon provide a refreshing zing.

Drinking this detox green juice regularly can help support your body's natural cleansing processes and provide an energy boost. Adjust the ingredient ratios to suit your taste preferences.

Beverages

6. Warm Lemon Water with Ginger

PreparationTime: 10 minutes

Juicing Time: 5 minutes

Total Time: 15 minutes

Serves: 1 (makes about 12 oz of juice)

- 2 cups kale, stems removed
- 1 cup spinach
- 1 green apple, cored
- 1 cucumber
- 1 inch piece fresh ginger, peeled
- 1 lemon, peeled

1. Wash all the produce thoroughly.

2. Run the kale, spinach, green apple, cucumber, ginger, and lemon through a juicer according to the manufacturer's Directions.

3. Stir or shake the juice to combine all the ingredients.

4. Pour the detox green juice into a glass and enjoy immediately.

This nutrient-dense green juice is packed with vitamins, minerals, and antioxidants from the leafy greens, apple, cucumber, ginger, and lemon. The ginger and lemon provide a refreshing zing.

Drinking this detox green juice regularly can help support your body's natural cleansing processes and provide an energy boost. Adjust the ingredient ratios to suit your taste preferences.

7. Coconut Water with Pineapple

PreparationTime: 5 minutes

Total Time: 5 minutes

Serves: 1

- 1 cup unsweetened coconut water
- 1/2 cup diced fresh pineapple

1. In a glass, combine the coconut water and diced pineapple.

2. Stir well to mix the ingredients together.

3. Serve immediately, over ice if desired.

The refreshing combination of coconut water and sweet pineapple makes this a delightful and hydrating beverage. Coconut water is naturally rich in electrolytes like potassium, making it an excellent choice for rehydrating after exercise or on a hot day.

The pineapple adds a tropical flavor and provides enzymes that can aid digestion. This simple drink is a great way to get in some extra vitamins, minerals, and antioxidants.

Feel free to adjust the ratio of coconut water to pineapple to suit your taste preferences. You can also blend the ingredients together for a smoothie-like consistency.

Enjoy this healthy and flavorful coconut water with pineapple!

Beverages

8. Iced Hibiscus Tea

PreparationTime: 10 minutes

Steep Time: 5-7 minutes

Chill Time: 2 hours

Total Time: 2 hours 15 minutes

Serves: 4 (makes 32 oz)

- 4 hibiscus tea bags or 4 tbsp dried hibiscus flowers
- 4 cups boiling water
- 2-3 tbsp honey or agave nectar (optional)
- Lemon slices for serving (optional)

1. In a heat-proof pitcher or teapot, steep the hibiscus tea bags or dried hibiscus flowers in the boiling water for 5-7 minutes.

2. Remove the tea bags or strain out the hibiscus flowers.

3. Stir in 2-3 tablespoons of honey or agave nectar, if desired, to sweeten the tea.

4. Allow the hibiscus tea to cool to room temperature, then refrigerate for at least 2 hours until completely chilled.

5. Serve the iced hibiscus tea over ice, garnished with lemon slices if desired.

The bright, tart, and slightly sweet flavor of hibiscus tea makes it a refreshing iced beverage. Hibiscus is rich in vitamin C, antioxidants, and has been linked to potential health benefits.

Adjust the sweetener amount to your taste preference. This iced hibiscus tea can be enjoyed year-round as a caffeine-free alternative to traditional iced tea.

Beverages

9. Matcha Latte with Almond Milk

PreparationTime: 5 minutes

Cook Time: 5 minutes

Total Time: 10 minutes

Serves: 1

- 1 cup unsweetened almond milk
- 1 tsp matcha green tea powder
- 1 tsp honey (optional)

1. In a small saucepan, heat the almond milk over medium heat, stirring frequently, until steaming hot but not boiling.

2. Remove the saucepan from the heat. Using a small whisk or milk frother, vigorously whisk the hot almond milk until it becomes frothy.

3. Sift the matcha green tea powder into the frothed almond milk and whisk again until the matcha is fully incorporated and the mixture is smooth.

4. If desired, stir in 1 tsp of honey to sweeten the matcha latte.

5. Pour the matcha latte into a mug and enjoy immediately while hot.

The combination of creamy almond milk and earthy, antioxidant-rich matcha creates a delicious and healthy latte. The frothing step adds a nice frothy texture.

You can adjust the amount of matcha powder to suit your taste preferences. This matcha latte makes a great alternative to coffee, providing a gentle caffeine boost along with numerous health benefits.

Beverages

10. Chia Fresca

PreparationTime: 5 minutes

Chilling Time: 30 minutes

Total Time: 35 minutes

Serves: 2

- 2 cups water
- 2 tbsp chia seeds
- 1 tbsp freshly squeezed lime juice
- 1 tbsp honey (or to taste)
- Lime slices for garnish (optional)

1. In a pitcher or large jar, combine the water and chia seeds. Stir well.

2. Cover and refrigerate for at least 30 minutes, stirring occasionally, to allow the chia seeds to swell and thicken the mixture.

3. Once thickened, stir in the lime juice and honey to taste. Start with 1 tbsp of honey and add more if desired.

4. Pour the chia fresca into glasses and garnish with lime slices, if using.

5. Serve chilled.

Chia fresca is a refreshing and hydrating drink made with chia seeds, lime, and honey. The chia seeds provide fiber, protein, and omega-3s, while the lime and honey add a bright, tangy-sweet flavor.

This drink is perfect for hot days or as a healthy alternative to sugary juices or sodas. The chia seeds also give it a fun, tapioca-like texture.

Feel free to adjust the amounts of lime juice and honey to suit your taste preferences. Enjoy this nutritious and delicious chia fresca!

Beverages

1. Vegan Lentil and Vegetable Stew

PreparationTime: 20 minutes

Cook Time: 45 minutes

Total Time: 1 hour 5 minutes

Serves: 4-6

- 1 tbsp olive oil
- 1 onion, diced
- 3 garlic cloves, minced
- 2 carrots, peeled and diced
- 2 celery stalks, diced
- 1 cup brown or green lentils, rinsed
- 4 cups vegetable broth
- 1 (14.5 oz) can diced tomatoes
- 2 tsp dried thyme
- 1 tsp dried oregano
- 1 bay leaf
- Salt and pepper to taste
- Chopped parsley for garnish (optional)

1. In a large pot or Dutch oven, heat the olive oil over medium heat. Add the onion and sauté for 5 minutes until translucent.

2. Add the garlic, carrots, and celery. Cook for 3-4 minutes, stirring frequently, until the vegetables start to soften.

3. Stir in the lentils, vegetable broth, diced tomatoes, thyme, oregano, and bay leaf. Season with salt and pepper.

4. Bring the stew to a boil, then reduce heat and let simmer for 35-40 minutes, until the lentils are tender.

5. Remove the bay leaf. Taste and adjust seasoning as needed.

6. Serve the lentil and vegetable stew hot, garnished with chopped parsley if desired. Enjoy with crusty bread.

This hearty, plant-based stew is packed with protein from the lentils and fiber from the vegetables. It's a comforting and nutritious meal.

Healthy One-Pot Meals

2. One-Pot Pasta Primavera

PreparationTime: 15 minutes
Cook Time: 20 minutes
Total Time: 35 minutes
Serves: 4

- 8 oz whole wheat pasta (such as penne or fusilli)
- 2 cups low-sodium vegetable broth
- 1 cup water
- 1 cup broccoli florets
- 1 cup sliced zucchini
- 1 cup halved cherry tomatoes
- 1/2 cup frozen peas
- 3 garlic cloves, minced
- 2 tbsp chopped fresh basil
- 2 tbsp grated Parmesan cheese (optional)
- Salt and pepper to taste

Healthy One-Pot Meals

1. In a large pot or Dutch oven, combine the uncooked pasta, vegetable broth, water, broccoli, zucchini, cherry tomatoes, and frozen peas.

2. Bring the mixture to a boil over high heat. Once boiling, reduce heat to medium-low and let simmer, stirring occasionally, for 12-15 minutes until the pasta is tender and the vegetables are cooked through.

3. Stir in the minced garlic and chopped basil. Cook for 2-3 more minutes.

4. Remove from heat and stir in the Parmesan cheese, if using. Season with salt and pepper to taste.

5. Serve the one-pot pasta primavera immediately, garnished with extra basil if desired.

This easy, one-pot pasta dish is loaded with fresh spring vegetables like broccoli, zucchini, and tomatoes. The pasta cooks right in the broth, making it a simple and flavorful meatless meal.

3. Vegan Chili with Sweet Potatoes

PreparationTime: 20 minutes

Cook Time: 45 minutes

Total Time: 1 hour 5 minutes

Serves: 4-6

- 1 tbsp olive oil
- 1 onion, diced
- 3 garlic cloves, minced
- 2 medium sweet potatoes, peeled and cubed
- 1 red bell pepper, diced
- 2 (15 oz) cans black beans, drained and rinsed
- 1 (15 oz) can kidney beans, drained and rinsed
- 1 (28 oz) can diced tomatoes
- 2 cups vegetable broth
- 2 tbsp chili powder
- 1 tsp ground cumin
- 1 tsp dried oregano
- 1/2 tsp smoked paprika
- Salt and pepper to taste
- Chopped cilantro for garnish (optional)

1. In a large pot or Dutch oven, heat the olive oil over medium heat. Add the onion and sauté for 5 minutes until translucent.

2. Add the garlic, sweet potatoes, and bell pepper. Cook for 3-4 minutes, stirring frequently.

3. Stir in the black beans, kidney beans, diced tomatoes, vegetable broth, chili powder, cumin, oregano, and smoked paprika. Season with salt and pepper.

4. Bring the chili to a boil, then reduce heat and let simmer for 35-40 minutes, until the sweet potatoes are tender.

5. Taste and adjust seasonings as needed.

6. Serve the vegan chili hot, garnished with chopped cilantro if desired. Enjoy with cornbread or tortilla chips.

The sweet potatoes add a delicious, natural sweetness to this hearty, plant-based chili. It's a comforting and nutritious meal.

Healthy One-Pot Meals

4. Moroccan Chickpea Stew

PreparationTime: 20 minutes

Cook Time: 45 minutes

Total Time: 1 hour 5 minutes

Serves: 4-6

- 2 tbsp olive oil
- 1 onion, diced
- 3 garlic cloves, minced
- 1 tbsp grated fresh ginger
- 2 tsp ground cumin
- 1 tsp ground coriander
- 1 tsp paprika
- 1/2 tsp ground cinnamon
- 1/4 tsp cayenne pepper (optional)
- 2 (15 oz) cans chickpeas, drained and rinsed
- 1 (14 oz) can diced tomatoes
- 2 cups vegetable broth
- 1 medium sweet potato, peeled and cubed
- 1 cup cauliflower florets
- 1 cup frozen peas
- Juice of 1 lemon
- Salt and pepper to taste
- Chopped cilantro for garnish (optional)

1. In a large pot or Dutch oven, heat the olive oil over medium heat. Add the onion and sauté for 5 minutes until translucent.

2. Stir in the garlic, ginger, cumin, coriander, paprika, cinnamon, and cayenne (if using). Cook for 1 minute until fragrant.

3. Add the chickpeas, diced tomatoes, vegetable broth, sweet potato, cauliflower, and frozen peas. Season with salt and pepper.

4. Bring the stew to a boil, then reduce heat and let simmer for 35-40 minutes, until the vegetables are tender.

5. Remove from heat and stir in the lemon juice.

6. Serve the Moroccan chickpea stew hot, garnished with chopped cilantro if desired. Enjoy with couscous or naan bread.

The blend of warm spices, chickpeas, and roasted vegetables creates a flavorful and comforting stew. It's a hearty, plant-based meal.

Healthy One-Pot Meals

5. Vegan Jambalaya

PreparationTime: 20 minutes

Cook Time: 45 minutes

Total Time: 1 hour 5 minutes

Serves: 4-6

- 1 tbsp olive oil
- 1 onion, diced
- 1 red bell pepper, diced
- 3 celery stalks, diced
- 3 garlic cloves, minced
- 1 cup uncooked long-grain white rice
- 1 (14 oz) can diced tomatoes
- 2 cups vegetable broth
- 1 tsp smoked paprika
- 1 tsp dried thyme
- 1 tsp dried oregano
- 1/2 tsp cayenne pepper (optional)
- 1 (15 oz) can kidney beans, drained and rinsed
- 1 (15 oz) can black-eyed peas, drained and rinsed
- Salt and pepper to taste
- Chopped green onions for garnish (optional)

Healthy One-Pot Meals

1. In a large pot or Dutch oven, heat the olive oil over medium heat. Add the onion, bell pepper, and celery. Sauté for 5-7 minutes until the vegetables are softened.

2. Stir in the garlic and cook for 1 minute until fragrant.

3. Add the uncooked rice, diced tomatoes, vegetable broth, smoked paprika, thyme, oregano, and cayenne (if using). Season with salt and pepper.

4. Bring the mixture to a boil, then reduce heat to low, cover, and simmer for 20-25 minutes, until the rice is tender.

5. Stir in the kidney beans and black-eyed peas. Cook for 5 more minutes to heat through.

6. Remove from heat and let stand, covered, for 5 minutes.

7. Fluff the jambalaya with a fork and serve hot, garnished with chopped green onions if desired.

This plant-based jambalaya is packed with Cajun-inspired flavors from the spices, vegetables, and beans. It's a hearty and satisfying one-pot meal.

Embracing a plant-based diet during menopause is a powerful way to support your health and well-being through this significant life transition. By focusing on whole, nutrient-dense foods, you can effectively manage symptoms such as hot flashes, night sweats, mood swings, and weight changes, while also promoting overall vitality.

Key Takeaways

1. Nourishing Your Body: A plant-based diet provides essential nutrients that are particularly beneficial during menopause. Phytoestrogens, calcium, vitamin D, omega-3 fatty acids, fiber, and antioxidants all play crucial roles in maintaining hormonal balance, bone health, heart health, and overall energy levels.

2. Delicious and Varied Meals: The recipes in this cookbook demonstrate that a plant-based diet can be both nutritious and delicious. From hearty breakfasts and satisfying lunches to flavorful dinners and indulgent desserts, there is no shortage of options to keep your meals exciting and enjoyable.

3. Ease of Transition: Adopting a plant-based diet doesn't have to be overwhelming. Starting gradually, planning your meals, experimenting with new recipes, focusing on whole foods, and staying hydrated are practical steps to help you make the switch smoothly.

Encouragement for the Journey Ahead

Menopause is a natural part of life, and navigating it with a focus on health and nutrition can make a significant difference in how you feel. The recipes and tips provided in this cookbook are designed to support you in making this transition as smooth and enjoyable as possible.

By choosing a plant-based diet, you are taking a proactive step towards better health and well-being. Enjoy the process of discovering new flavors, nourishing your body, and feeling your best during this important phase of life.

Thank you for joining me on this culinary journey. May your kitchen be filled with vibrant, plant-based meals that bring you joy, health, and balance during menopause and beyond.